Applied Social Science for Nursing Students

Mark Molesworth
Iain Atherton

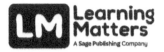

Learning Matters
A Sage Publishing Company
1 Oliver's Yard
55 City Road
London EC1Y 1SP

Sage Publications Inc.
2455 Teller Road
Thousand Oaks, California 91320

Sage Publications India Pvt Ltd
B 1/I 1 Mohan Cooperative Industrial Area
Mathura Road
New Delhi 110 044

Sage Publications Asia-Pacific Pte Ltd
3 Church Street
#10-04 Samsung Hub
Singapore 049483

Editor: Martha Cunneen
Development editors: Lyndsay Oliver and Ruth Lilly
Senior project editor: Chris Marke
Project management: Westchester Publishing
Services UK
Marketing Manager: Ruslana Khatagova
Cover design: Sheila Tong
Typeset by: C&M Digitals (P) Ltd, Chennai, India
Printed in the UK

© Mark Molesworth and Iain Atherton, 2024

Apart from any fair dealing for the purposes of
research or private study, or criticism or review, as
permitted under the Copyright, Designs and Patents
Act, 1988, this publication may be reproduced, stored
or transmitted in any form, or by any means, only with
the prior permission in writing of the publishers, or in
the case of reprographic reproduction, in accordance
with the terms of licences issued by the Copyright
Licensing Agency. Enquiries concerning reproduction
outside those terms should be sent to the publishers.
Crown Copyright material is published with the
permission of the controller of HMSO.

Library of Congress Control Number: 2023944524

British Library Cataloguing in Publication Data

A catalogue record for this book is available from the
British Library

ISBN 978-1-5297-9704-6
ISBN 978-1-5297-9703-9 (pbk)

At Sage we take sustainability seriously. Most of our products are printed in the UK using responsibly sourced
papers and boards. When we print overseas we ensure sustainable papers are used as measured by the Paper
Chain Project grading system. We undertake an annual audit to monitor our sustainability.

Contents

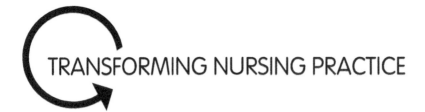

TRANSFORMING NURSING PRACTICE

Transforming Nursing Practice is a series tailor made for pre-registration student nurses. Each book in the series is:

- Affordable
- Mapped to the NMC Standards of proficiency for registered nurses
- Full of active learning features
- Focused on applying theory to practice

Each book addresses a core topic and they have been carefully developed to be simple to use, quick to read and written in clear language.

An invaluable series of books that explicitly relates to the NMC standards. Each book covers a different topic that students need to explore in order to develop into a qualified nurse... I would recommend this series to all Pre-Registered nursing students whatever their field or year of study.

LINDA ROBSON,
Senior Lecturer at Edge Hill University

Many titles in the series are on our recommended reading list and for good reason - the content is up to date and easy to read. These are the books that actually get used beyond training and into your nursing career.

EMMA LYDON,
Adult Student Nursing

ABOUT THE SERIES EDITORS

DR MOOI STANDING is an Independent Nursing Consultant (UK and International) and is responsible for the core knowledge, adult nursing and personal and professional learning skills titles. She is an experienced NMC Quality Assurance Reviewer of educational programmes and a Professional Regulator Panellist on the NMC Practice Committee. Mooi is also Board member of Special Olympics Malaysia, enabling people with intellectual disabilities to participate in sports and athletics nationally and internationally.

DR SANDRA WALKER is a Clinical Academic in Mental Health working between Southern Health Trust and the University of Southampton and responsible for the mental health nursing titles. She is a Qualified Mental Health Nurse with a wide range of clinical experience spanning more than 25 years.

BESTSELLING TEXTBOOKS

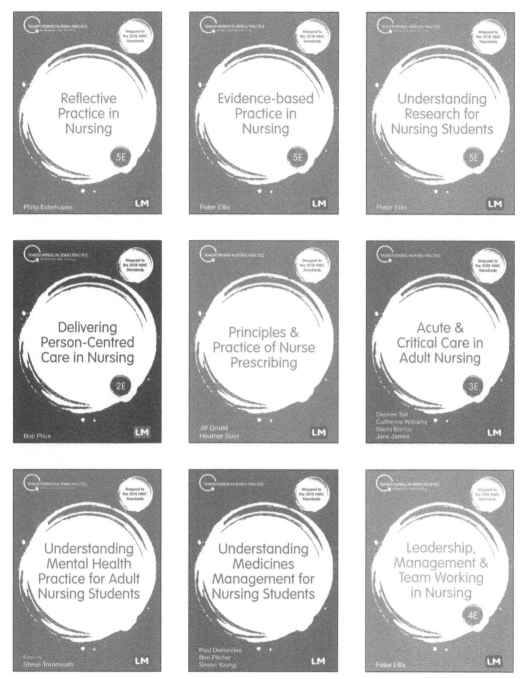

You can find a full list of textbooks in the *Transforming Nursing Practice* series at

https://uk.sagepub.com/TNP-series

Acknowledgements

Iain would like to thank:

First and foremost, my co-author, Mark. His knowledge of social science teaching in nursing, demonstrated through his brilliant PhD, and dynamic and creative thinking have both made this book possible and made the journey one of personal learning. To all our colleagues at Sage: Ruth, Martha and Lyndsay. My colleagues in the Pedagogical Matters group, whose passion for nurse education and population health is always enthusing. The seminar series their funding made possible (ES/L000741/1) has contributed enormously to this book.

Finally, to Laura, Tom and Rachel for their constant fun, patience and support.

Mark would like to thank:

My co-author, Iain, for his enduring wisdom, patience and expertise while we wrote the book together. Thanks to the editorial team at Sage, including Ruth, Martha and Lyndsay, and the anonymous reviewers. I would also like to recognise the contribution of students who participated in the research that has greatly informed the book.

A special thank you to Amber, Harry, Cora and Bodhi for their love and understanding throughout the long journey of writing this book.

About the authors

Dr Iain Atherton is a reader in nursing and population health at Edinburgh Napier University. After qualifying as a registered general nurse, he practised in various areas, including neurology, and for an aid organisation in Romania before reading for a degree in development studies, a broad ranging social sciences degree. After gaining a master's degree in medical demography at the London School of Hygiene and Tropical Medicine, and completing a doctorate at the University of St Andrews, he has advanced to an academic career. He has developed and run modules on population health for practice, research methods and statistical analysis. He is a co-director of the Economic and Social Research Council (ESRC)-funded Scottish Centre for Administrative Data Research, where he uses linked administrative and census data to answer key policy relevant questions. His research has covered areas including inequalities in cancer survival, increased home deaths during the COVID-19 pandemic, and population perspectives towards care in the last days of life. He is dad to two children, with whom he enjoys interrailing to far-flung corners of Europe.

Mark Molesworth is a registered nurse and senior lecturer based in Scotland. He is Programme Leader for BSc/BSc (Hons) Nursing Studies (all fields) at Glasgow Caledonian University. Mark has a wealth of experience within different care settings, including nursing in the Royal Air Force, the Scottish Prison Service and acute NHS services. He is passionate about nurse education and supporting students to develop critical understanding across theory and practice. His PhD explored student nurses' experiences of the social sciences and biosciences during their studies. Mark has three children and enjoys family camping trips.

Introduction

About this book

In a complex and rapidly evolving world, student nurses and other health professionals must be flexible, adaptive and creative. Inclusive and systemic perspectives are necessary to understand and respond to local and global health needs. This book builds upon the wealth of insights offered by the social sciences to improve your ability to provide effective care in the modern world. Nursing that draws on the social sciences understands that care is often individualised but occurs within a highly influential set of socio-economic circumstances. Recognising the needs of people, communities and populations requires nurses to draw upon concepts from the social science disciplines.

This book will introduce you to a variety of theoretical frameworks, techniques and case studies. Applying social sciences to nursing will show how it can support effective and compassionate care. It will help you to recognise the influences behind the holistic care needs of individuals and how these can be met. In addition, you will learn why cultural competency is important and how to incorporate it into your daily work. In doing so, you will improve your ability to recognise and challenge forms of discrimination and inequalities that impact under-represented groups.

Healthcare policy and social transformation are influenced by activism and politics. Whether through community organising, lobbying or seeking policy reform, student nurses play an important role in bringing about positive change. This book will provide a grasp of the political landscape and the power dynamics, exploring how you and your patients can have a voice in shaping the future of healthcare. We hope you will find the text a valuable resource in using understanding from the social sciences to make a meaningful difference in the lives of the patients and communities to whom you provide care. Use this book to help navigate towards a more thoughtful, compassionate and transformative approach to healthcare.

Requirements for the NMC Standards of Proficiency for Registered Nurses

The Nursing and Midwifery Council (NMC) has established standards of proficiency to be met by applicants to different parts of the register, and these are the standards it considers necessary for safe and effective practice. This book is structured so that it will help you to understand and meet the proficiencies required for entry to the NMC register. The relevant proficiencies are presented at the start of each chapter so that you can clearly see which ones the chapter addresses. The proficiencies have been designed to be generic so apply to all fields of nursing and all care settings. This is because all nurses must be able to meet the needs of any person they encounter in their practice, regardless of their stage of life or health challenges, whether these are mental, physical, cognitive or behavioural.

This book includes the latest standards for 2018 onwards, taken from *Future nurse: standards of proficiency for registered nurses* (NMC, 2018b).

Learning features

Learning by reading text is not always easy. Therefore, each chapter contains a range of activities, scenarios and case studies. These interactive learning tools provide a more immersive and practical experience, bridging the gap between academic theory and real-life circumstances. They can build critical thinking and problem-solving abilities by reviewing the exercises and scenarios, while case studies provide insights into how you might approach different circumstances. The activities will help you comprehend the topics being discussed and better prepare you for real-world nursing practice.

We have also included 'Student Voices', which share real experiences from student nurses regarding how the social sciences are relevant to their practice. These perspectives were collected during Mark Molesworth's PhD inquiry exploring how the disciplines feature within nurse education. You will also be introduced to Bernadette and Abigail, two fictional nursing students who become friends and whose experiences are threaded throughout the book. Each time you revisit the pair, you will be encouraged to think about how key concepts being explored in the chapter apply to their circumstances. In addition, all the activities that feature a question will have possible answers at the relevant chapter's end. This will enable you to compare your responses to see if they are similar to those of the authors.

Chapter 1 Social science informed nursing

Chapter aims

By the end of this chapter, you should be able to:

- briefly describe what the social sciences involve;
- outline the origins of the social sciences;
- discuss ways in which sociology and psychology can support nursing practice;
- recognise complexities regarding the social sciences and how they relate to nursing.

Introduction

This chapter will provide you with insights into what the social sciences involve and how they can benefit the nursing profession. It will consider the limitations of relying too heavily upon personal experience, highlighting how information from the social sciences can support your nursing practice. The chapter includes a brief introduction to the social sciences and their origins before the discussion moves on to focus on their relevance to nursing. We touch on some of the complexities and controversies surrounding the relationship between the nursing profession, including a critical review of the Eurocentric nature of the nursing curriculum. We hope that you will find the social sciences are an accessible and exciting part of your learning journey during this chapter.

Setting the scene

Have you ever wondered how people can see a particular situation differently from yourself despite it appearing so obvious? This might be related to different views on a social or political situation, or perhaps an issue that has come up during your nursing studies. Despite having the potential to be surprising or even frustrating and confusing, the reasons behind these differing perspectives can become more understandable when we explore why they exist. We are all individuals who have lived different lives, sometimes dramatically so. These lived histories, integrated with other factors such as our cognitive make-up, help to shape how we uniquely perceive the world around us.

The unique perspective you bring to the profession can help inform your practice and connect with others. There is a lot of value in nurses drawing upon their past experiences and beliefs. However, if we relied entirely on our personal experience, this would limit our ability to develop a deeper understanding of the contexts and people we care for. Learning about the perspectives and experiences of others can take us beyond the limitations of relying on personal experience. This can be gained by carefully listening to the people we care for. This is also where the social sciences can be of benefit to every nurse. Together they provide a wealth of information and evidence that can enable nurses to look beyond their own experiences to understand better the people and communities they work with.

The social sciences often draw upon established theories and frameworks to support this work. Each discipline has its own set of theories, models and ideas that help orientate its worldview. A worldview can be defined as the collection of attitudes, values and understandings about the world around us (Gray, 2011). This means that how a sociologist looks at an interaction between a nurse and a patient in a hospital ward will likely differ from how a psychologist would look at the same situation. We all have our worldview, a kind of lens through which we understand the world. Our worldview informs every thought and behaviour that we have. Through practice and research activity, each social science discipline provides differing perspectives and insights concerning the world. These can help to inform our worldview, broadening and deepening our perception of the world around us.

Activity 1.1   Reflection

Think about your worldview on the role of nursing in society. Write down some of the factors that have contributed to and shaped your unique worldview. This might include family, friends, life experiences, interests, etc. Consider how this might differ from the perspective of your fellow student nurses.

An outline answer is given at the end of the chapter.

Over recent decades, there have been rapid and dramatic changes in society. These have been accelerated through global events and the proliferation of digital and communication technologies. The social sciences have constantly evolved to provide insights into our changing world. At the same time, they provide opportunities to imagine and move towards alternative futures. Social scientists undertake research and develop theories that help us understand ourselves and the world around us. This is important at an individual level as it allows people to look beyond their personal experiences and be more sensitive to the lived experiences of others, as well as the privileges and barriers that may have impacted their life. As outlined in the book's introduction, the disciplines of sociology and psychology are the social sciences that are the most relevant for nursing. Let's explore what these two disciplines incorporate.

What are sociology and psychology?

We begin this discussion by looking at sociology. Sociology is a broad social science discipline that embraces many aspects of human activity (British Sociological Association, 2022). It can be defined as *the study of social life, social change and the social causes and consequences of human behaviour* (American Sociological Association, 2019, page 1). Sociologists investigate the structure of groups, organisations and societies and how people interact within these contexts. Many educators would like to ensure nurses develop sociological understanding and awareness (e.g. Atherton and Kyle, 2014; Davies, 2012; Goodman and Grant, 2017; Koch et al., 2016; Lipscomb, 2017; Matthews, 2015a).

By applying a sociological lens, nurses can use sociology to critically explore, understand and improve their contexts and practices. This means using sociological concepts and theories and applying these to an area of interest. It has been argued that the sociological lens is more vital to the nursing profession than ever before (Doherty et al., 2013; Forrest, 2016). One of the reasons for this is how it can help you understand current societal challenges. For example, your community placements may allow you to use the sociological lens to explore the nurse's role in recognising and addressing increasing inequalities within society (Edgley, Timmons and Crosbie, 2009, page 20; Harris and Nimmo, 2013). You might apply a sociological lens to explore how inequalities impact a community where you are undertaking one of your placements. Carol's placement with the Health Visiting Service in a deprived area in Scotland provided her with this type of opportunity (see Student Voices: Carol). Please note that most Student Voices boxes are adapted from a research project by one of this book's authors into nursing students' experiences of sociology and psychology during their studies.

Student voices: Carol

My Practice Supervisor and I talked about employment, we talked about lack of lifestyle opportunities, that there are very few resources put into an area that could really use them, we talked about a lack of education opportunities.

Carol, 2nd Year Adult Student Nurse

Activity 1.2   Critical thinking

Thinking about Carol's point in the previous Student Voices box, why are employment and education opportunities significant from a health perspective?

An outline answer is given at the end of the chapter.

Like sociology, psychology is interested in understanding human beings, although its focus is on individual thought and behaviour. The name psychology is derived from the Greek words *psyche* (the human soul, mind or spirit) and *logos* (meaning knowledge, discourse or study) (Gross, 2020). NHS Health Education England (2023, page 1) describes psychology as *the scientific study of the mind and how it dictates and influences our behaviour, from communication and memory to thought and emotion.* Psychology is a diverse discipline that explores many aspects of human experience, often focusing on thought processes and behaviour. From a nursing perspective, an understanding of psychology assists with recognising the factors that impact individual and group behaviour. As a nurse, you can use this knowledge when providing care to respond to behaviours while supporting individuals to make positive changes in their lives, particularly in mental and physical health. Here Simon explains his experiences related to psychology while on placement.

Student voices: Simon

I had the opportunity to sit in with the pre-operative assessment and counsel people on their fears and anxieties when they came for their surgery. It made me think about the psychological aspects of undergoing a surgical operation.

Simon, 1st Year Adult Student Nurse

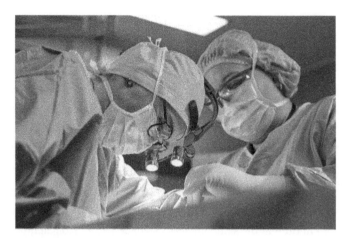

Figure 1.1 A patient undergoing surgery

Source: Georgii – stock.adobe.com

Activity 1.3   Reflection

Read Simon's experiences in the previous Student Voices box and then answer the following question.

Consider the psychological aspects of waiting to undergo a surgical operation, such as the one in Figure 1.1.

What do you think would be the benefits of this learning experience for Simon's nursing practice?

An outline answer is given at the end of the chapter.

We have begun to explore how the social sciences can play an essential role in your nursing practice. However, it is worth being aware that the social sciences consist of different perspectives. A significant part of developing new knowledge and understanding within the social sciences arises through debate and disagreement. Unlike other disciplines, such as human biology, there are rarely clear-cut and universally accepted ideas within the social sciences. However, scratch beneath the surface and seemingly settled theory is often debated in the other disciplines. The contested nature of the social sciences can be disconcerting for someone unfamiliar with this arena. Please don't be put off by this. Taking a critical approach and debating different ideas can provide new insights while helping to highlight assumptions and misconceptions. As you become more familiar with the social sciences, you can adopt a similar approach during your studies, perhaps while reading different pieces of research on a topic. It will help you explore other ideas, gradually becoming more critical and thoughtful about your nursing practice and the world around you.

Case study: Bernadette and Abigail

Bernadette and Abigail are two student nurses who started their nurse education together at the same university. Bernadette recently moved to the UK from her extended family home in Paris to study. She was born in Nigeria and moved to Europe with her parents when she was a toddler. Bernadette still has many friends and family in Paris and speaks to them most days. Bernadette is unsure where she wants to work once she has finished her studies in the UK.

Meanwhile, Abigail grew up locally and has always lived at her mum's house, a short bus ride from the university. Her mum is a carer and works with older adults with disabilities. Abigail wants to work at the regional hospital when she finishes her nurse education. They are both single mothers with young children at the same nursery. Bernadette and Abigail quickly become close friends while studying on the nursing programme.

Activity 1.4   Reflection

How may Bernadette and Abigail's experiences shape how they approach their nursing studies?

An outline answer is given at the end of the chapter.

Before we explore some of the insights provided by the social sciences, it is helpful to review how the disciplines originated. This provides a backdrop to the contributions they have made and also helps to define their specific areas of interest.

Social science origins

This section will briefly set out historical developments related to the origins of sociology and psychology. It will help you understand how the disciplines came into being and thus provide context for some of the theories and ideas relevant to nurses' work. You will be introduced to key individuals and dates, but do not worry about trying to remember all the details. It may be more worthwhile to think about how the developments relate to the emergence of nursing within the UK. Nursing developed during the 1800s through the work of pioneers such as Florence Nightingale and Mary-Jane Seacole. It finally became a registered profession with the passing of the Nurses' Registration Act in 1919. As you read through this section, you may see that sociology and psychology evolved during a similar period.

Activity 1.5 Evidence-based practice and research

To learn more about the development of nursing registration within the UK, please read the following article in the *Nursing Times* by Sheperd (2019): Timeline: the road to nurse registration in the UK.

In which year did the NMC become the regulator for the nursing profession?

An outline answer is given at the end of the chapter.

Before we move on, it is essential to be aware that enquiry related to sociology and psychology did not arise spontaneously in the West; it grew out of many years of philosophical thought about society and individual people and their behaviours. For example, the ancient Greeks were interested in the structures and functioning of society. As a discipline, sociology emerged in Europe around the end of the industrial revolution and towards the late 1800s. Auguste Comte (1798–1857) is often considered the founding father of sociology. He is also credited with the first use of the term 'sociology' in 1838, although it had been in use before this date. Émile Durkheim (1858–1917), and other prominent figures such as Karl Marx (1818–83) and Max Weber (1864–1920), firmly established sociology as an important field of inquiry and theoretical development. In the next chapter, we'll look at how two key approaches within sociology are associated with these early theorists: functionalism and conflict theory. However, this is only part of the story of the development of sociology.

Murji, Neal and Solomos (2022) point out that the origin story of sociology has often overlooked the contribution of key individuals. This is particularly the case for people from groups who traditionally had limited opportunities to work in the field of sociology and other academic disciplines. These include Harriet Martineau (1802–76), sometimes described as the first woman sociologist, and WEB Du Bois (1868–1963), an American sociologist and civil rights activist. Another example is the earlier work of Ibn Khaldun (1332–1406), a Muslim scholar who wrote widely regarding sociological topics.

Activity 1.6 Team working

Social scientists work in a wide variety of areas, including academic, professional and policy settings. Can you think of an example of a specific role for each area?

An outline answer is given at the end of the chapter.

Psychology also has broad roots underpinning its emergence as a discipline. The seventeenth-century French philosopher René Descartes provided a new understanding of psychological phenomena. He was engaged in understanding the relations between emotions, reason and the brain (Kirkebøen, 2019). Descartes expressed the famous statement: *I think, therefore I am* (in Latin: *cogito, ergo sum*). Through this phrase, Descartes is claiming that the very act of doubting his existence irrefutably proved his existence. This type of philosophical certainty is rare. Later developments built upon philosophical ideas related to human thought and behaviour. This was accompanied by an increasing interest in the use of observation and measurement to advance knowledge.

Concept summary: Empirical inquiry

Empirical inquiry is focused on generating knowledge through observation and experimentation. It purports to be objective in its techniques and relies upon establishing and investigating measurable aspects of a phenomenon. It uses research methods that can be replicated, which helps in the process of validating any findings.

The development of these empirical approaches (see the Concept Summary box) took a significant step forward when Wilhelm Wundt's experimental psychology laboratory was recognised as an institute by Leipzig University, Germany, in 1879. Indeed, this is the date often given as when scientific psychology was founded (Green, 2021). Wundt used experimental equipment and techniques to examine mental processes, observing and analysing the fundamental structures of thought and perception (Gross, 2020). These early developments in the field of psychology were concerned with the empirical aspects of psychology. Over time these were joined by alternative perspectives, such as the psychodynamic approach and behaviourism. The psychodynamic approach arose from Sigmund Freud's (1858–1939) work to understand the mind and our unconscious's influence on everyday behaviour.

Behaviouristic psychology is an approach that focuses on observable behaviour. We'll pick up on aspects of these approaches and their relevance to holistic nursing care within Chapter 3. Another significant development was humanistic psychology, which arose in America during the 1950s, which we will consider in more detail within the next chapter. Now that you better understand the social sciences and their origins, it is time to look at their relevance to nursing in more detail.

The social sciences in nursing

The Willis Commission (Royal College of Nursing (RCN), 2012) established that practical learning must be underpinned by relevant knowledge from the social science disciplines. Current standards for nurse education require that your nurse education include theoretical instruction, including the social sciences, inclusive of sociology and psychology (NMC, 2018a). However, the social science disciplines and their historical developments may seem distant from the nursing practice you encounter during your placements. You might hear some people say that nursing is mainly practical, asking why learning from other academic disciplines is necessary. In the following paragraphs, we will counter these views by providing examples of how the social sciences are relevant to your nursing practice.

Nurses work with people from every background during their careers, agreeing and providing care that meets their individual needs. The social sciences are a crucial aspect of nursing knowledge by providing research and theoretical frameworks that assist in exploring social contexts. These can expose you to fascinating insights into how others perceive and act in the world. As a nurse, this is crucial to recognise the circumstances and needs of the people to whom you provide care. An example of how this may apply is provided in the following scenario.

Scenario: Recognising circumstances and needs

Imagine you are on a six-week placement working in a health centre in prison. During the placement, you are working alongside your Practice Supervisor to support the health and wellbeing of prisoners. This involves many different roles, such as providing a daily clinic for prisoners with health concerns, administering medications, liaising with other healthcare professionals and attending medical emergencies. Different wings within the prison separate prisoners according to the length of sentence or type of conviction.

Your family was worried about any risks associated with being on placement in prison. You feel nervous the first few days going up to the large gates and through the reception area into the prison, but soon the nerves start to fade. Over time you begin to get to know some prisoners as you work alongside your Practice Supervisor, hearing aspects of their life stories. Before you came into the prison, you had preconceptions that most people in jail were all terrible people because of their crimes. Throughout the placement, you begin to realise that the situation is more complex than you first thought. You find that many of the prisoners had difficult life circumstances prior to their crimes, and most are engaged in employment and education activities within the prison to try to improve their life upon release. You are surprised to find that you get on well in the setting and enjoy supporting the prisoners alongside your Practice Supervisor.

Your Practice Supervisor highlights some of the work that has been undertaken by social scientists, which shows that prisoners are more likely to suffer mental health issues. You also learn that a large proportion of those are from disadvantaged communities, with Black people being over-represented within the prison population (Ministry of Justice, 2021). On one of the days, your Practice Supervisor organises for you to speak with the prison psychologist and sit in on a consultation with a prisoner whom you have been supporting. The prisoner

(Continued)

consents to this. You hear that the individual had been a victim of a crime earlier in their life, and observe the psychologist helping them plan strategies to deal with triggers related to their past traumas.

By the end of the placement, you realise that nursing is about far more than providing practical care. You feel you have a better understanding of how a person's circumstances can affect their physical and mental health and vice versa. Your Practice Assessor is impressed by your skills and highlights your non-judgemental approach within the placement assessment feedback. You're not sure if you would like to work as a nurse in prison once registered, but you have learned many things that will benefit you in your future career.

Activity 1.7   Decision-making

1. What are two ways that you can use to adopt a non-judgemental approach if providing care in a prison setting?
2. Consider the psychological issues that may come with being a prisoner. Write down the ways these may affect mental health.

An outline answer is given at the end of the chapter.

Sociology and psychology support nurses in bridging the biomedical with behavioural and social elements of health (McPherson, 2008). Person-centred care has been highlighted as the 'golden thread' that runs through all pre-registration nursing education (RCN, 2012). Chapman (2017) describes person-centred care as developing an understanding of each person as an individual and involving them in decisions about their care. It is important to understand the situation from their perspective while tak-

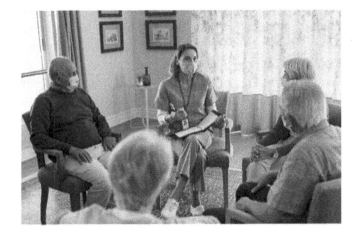

Figure 1.2   A nurse consults with residents about the service

Source: Rido – stock.adobe.com

ing into account their ideas, wishes and interests. It can also involve seeking input from service users on how the services they use are shaped and delivered, as shown in Figure 1.2. The concept of patient-centred care, familiar to all nurses, has roots that can be traced back to the developments within social sciences (Percy and Richardson, 2018). When asked, student nurses themselves recognise the social sciences as providing the context of health that can prompt them to question their values and prejudices.

For example, Mowforth, Harrison and Morris (2005, page 45) asked nursing students about their experiences with psychology and sociology during their studies, with one of the participants providing the following response:

> *They have helped me look at myself and question my values, and what has really surprised me is I did not realise how prejudiced I was, but studying psychology and sociology has really opened my eyes and its come to a point now where I think I have had to change my attitudes really. It has been quite painful.*

Understanding developed through the social sciences can influence the way you interact in practice settings, as experienced by Gary when supporting patients with complex backgrounds in an acute setting (see Student Voices: Gary). Nurses risk limiting their ability to provide tailored care if they do not account for the factors that influence a person's thoughts and behaviours. By adopting a non-judgemental approach, you can learn more about people and develop greater awareness of the facilitators and barriers that impact health.

Student voices: Gary

> *Mentally stopping yourself from making snap judgements about people and almost taking a mental breath and a bit of space before you actually deal with people.*

Gary, 1st Year Adult Nursing Student

Activity 1.8   Decision-making

Read Gary's point in the previous Student Voices box and then answer the following questions:

1. What are some of the problems with making snap judgements about people you are caring for?
2. Why might it be helpful to use non-judgemental approaches with a patient that you do not know?

An outline answer is given at the end of the chapter.

In the previous sections, we have introduced you to the value that the social sciences offer the nursing profession. However, it is worth being aware that the relationship between the disciplines and social science is complex. As mentioned earlier, some question the value that academic disciplines can offer a practice-based profession. There are ongoing debates regarding the relevance of the social sciences to nursing students and the extent to which they should be incorporated into your studies (Molesworth and Lewitt, 2019). This is partly due to the sometimes tense relationship between the disciplines and the nursing profession, particularly in the case of sociology.

Sociology has a long history of examining and critiquing the construction and role of professions, including nursing. These inquiries fall within what may be considered a 'sociology *of* nursing', in contrast to the 'sociology *for* nursing' that we are focused on in this book. They explore controversial issues, such as whether nursing should be considered a profession or not (Ayala, 2020). Although some of the topics that the sociology of nursing addresses can be complex, they provide a useful outside perspective on the roles and structure of the nursing profession. For example, Snee, White and Cox's (2020) analysis highlights nostalgic views of the nurse within the public imagination and how gendered ways of viewing nursing endure. An issue we touch on in various points within the book, the under-representation of women in leadership positions for example (see Chapter 5). Now that you appreciate some of the complexities in the relationship between nursing and social science, the next section will focus on a particularly relevant aspect of the nursing curriculum that the social sciences can help us explore.

The nursing curriculum

One crucial area of critique regarding nursing education relates to Eurocentrism. This refers to privileging of Western voices, knowledge and customs within higher education (Baumgartner and Johnson-Bailey, 2008). It is linked to issues of racism and the need for nursing curricula to be more culturally diverse (Nairn et al., 2012). These issues reflect broader problems within the nursing profession, such as nurses of African-Caribbean heritage experiencing workplace bias and undermining cultural identities for 'Eurocentric' ideas of professionalism (Allen, 2021). Additionally, racism is experienced through structural biases, such as the over-representation of Black nurses within disciplinary procedures (Archibong et al., 2019) or through the behaviours and attitudes of colleagues and patients (Etowa, 2016).

Research summary: Anti-racism on campus

The Equality and Human Rights Commission (2019) published a report tackling racial harassment within higher education. It highlighted that almost a quarter of students from minority ethnic backgrounds said they had experienced racial harassment since starting their course, including physical attacks, racist jokes, racist insults, microaggressions and exclusion. Similar experiences were recounted by more than a quarter of staff. These experiences can severely affect mental health, educational outcomes and career progression (Universities UK, 2020). Advance HE (2020) is an influential charitable organisation that works to improve higher education for staff, students and society. They have devised the Advance HE Declaration on Anti-Racism while also providing resources to help Scottish Universities tackle racism on campus.

One area of focus within the work of Advance HE is the Anti-Racist Curriculum Project. Glasgow Caledonian University is an example of an institution taking forward developments in this area. It has established a group working in partnership with students to decolonise the curriculum, identifying systems and structures that are unrepresentative, inaccessible and privileged in nature (Campbell, 2022). The group's activities extend to the nursing department and its work to identify and tackle racism within the formal, informal and hidden curriculum. Whether you are studying in Scotland or elsewhere, we hope you will find that your university is taking steps to address racism.

Activity 1.9   Critical thinking

Look on your university's website to see if you find any information regarding measures they are taking to promote anti-racism.

An outline answer is given at the end of the chapter.

You and your university can play an essential role in reducing discrimination and promoting inclusion within the nursing curriculum and the wider profession. Many nurse education departments are trying to achieve this by forming diversity, equity and inclusion committees (Zappas et al., 2021). With student involvement, these could be used to develop strategies to promote diversity within the content and teaching approaches within programmes, tied in with other measures being taken by your university, the NHS and other organisations involved in nurse education. Read through Research Summary: Anti-Racism on Campus for an example of this type of development. We'll look in more detail at how you can get more involved in promoting anti-racism within nursing during Chapter 5.

Chapter summary

This chapter has introduced you to the social sciences and the key disciplines we focus on in this book. You have learned what the social sciences involve and a brief history of

(Continued)

their origins. The chapter has explored how sociology and psychology can help you to inform and develop your nursing practice. It is evident through the discussion that the social sciences continually evolve with new and competing perspectives coming forward. The resulting knowledge is useful for understanding the nursing profession and the people and communities nurses provide care to. However, it can also be disconcerting for someone looking for clear-cut answers. The chapter has also explored how the social sciences can help to expose difficult issues that the nursing profession must continue to address, such as Eurocentrism and racism. Now you have this information, the rest of the book will detail specific theoretical and research-based knowledge from the social sciences that can further support your development as a nursing student.

Activities: Brief outline answers

Activity 1.1   Reflection

Perhaps your worldview of nursing is influenced by the care you or a relative have previously received from nurses. This will further depend upon the country where you received the care and your preconceptions of nurses. These preconceptions will likely have been influenced by information online and perhaps through media such as TV programmes you have watched.

Activity 1.2   Critical thinking

Education and employment opportunities are important factors in health outcomes. People's health is directly affected by education because it informs them about healthier lifestyle choices and the importance of preventative care. On the other hand, employment provides financial stability while also reducing stress, which is a known factor in various health issues. Employment can indirectly impact health by influencing people's living conditions, diet and mental well-being. You will be responsible for patients whose health may be influenced by their level of education and employment status. You can become a more effective nurse by recognising these important social determinants of health.

Activity 1.3   Reflection

The opportunity for Simon to learn about the fears and anxieties of patients undergoing surgery is likely to benefit his practice in several ways. It will give him insight into the communication styles and types of information that can help patients address any uncertainties they have about going into surgery. The experience may highlight the importance of actively listening to the patient to find out how they feel about the surgery. This can help Simon better understand why sedatives may sometimes be used to alleviate fear and anxiety the night before or in the time leading up to the surgery. Simon's learning from the pre-assessment clinic will assist him to recognise why undergoing surgery can often be both a mentally and physically challenging experience, informing how he supports patients on admission and during the post-operative period.

Activity 1.4   Reflection

They have several things in common, which may mean they approach their nursing programme in a similar manner, for example, juggling being a busy parent with their studies and other responsibilities. However, their lived histories are likely to mean some cultural differences, and their conceptions of healthcare may vary.

Activity 1.5   Evidence-based practice and research

1.   The NMC became the regulator for nursing within the UK in 2002.

Activity 1.6   Team working

- Academic – social science lecturer; researcher.
- Professional – psychologist; media analyst.
- Policy – adviser; statistician.

Activity 1.7   Decision-making

1.   To adopt a non-judgemental approach, you should treat all people with dignity and respect regardless of their circumstances. This will ensure your practice is aligned with the NMC (2018c) *Code of professional standards.*

2.   There are many answers here. Concerns about family outside of the prison and having limitations on life choices may bring stressors. Worrying about release and stigmatisation from society and employers may cause anxiety.

Activity 1.8   Decision-making

Snap judgements are based on limited information. Inaccurate assessments of a patient's health status, needs and preferences can lead to ineffective or harmful treatment plans. Unconscious biases and stereotypes can influence snap judgements. A healthcare professional may assume a patient's lifestyle, behaviour or compliance based on age, race, ethnicity, socio-economic status, etc. This affects care quality and health disparities. Additionally, snap judgements can impede patient–provider communication and damage therapeutic relationships.

By displaying non-judgemental care, you can learn more about the patient and their situation. This can improve patient assessment. Understanding a patient improves outcomes and satisfaction. Non-judgemental care allows healthcare providers to recognise and challenge their biases and stereotypes. This improves care and reduces health disparities leading to an enhanced therapeutic relationship.

Activity 1.9   Critical thinking

1.   You should find that there is information about anti-racism online. If you don't find anything, try searching for discrimination instead to see what the university has published on the topic. If you still cannot find any relevant information, why not discuss it with one of your lecturers to see if they can point you in the right direction.

2.   Employment and education are important aspects of having access to good health. Being unemployed or having a reduced level of education has been shown to influence health outcomes negatively.

Further reading

Chapman H (2017) Nursing theories 1: person-centred care. *Nursing Times* [online]; 113: 10, 59.

Hazel Chapman's article provides a detailed discussion regarding person-centred care and its theoretical origins. This will be useful preparation for the next chapter, where we explore the topic in more detail.

Etowa J (2016) Diversity, racism and eurocentric-normative practice in healthcare. *International Journal of Health Sciences and Research*, 6(1): 278–289.

Review this article to gain an interesting and, at times, upsetting insight into the experiences of nurses from a minority background. Although the study was based in Canada, it has many learning points for nurses across the West.

Molesworth, M and Lewitt, M (2019) Sociology in UK nurse education curricula: a review of the literature from 1919–2019. *Social Theory and Health*, 17: 427–442.

Review this article for a detailed insight into the development of the relationship between sociology and nurse education. This extensive article sets out key milestones in the relationship from the Nurses' Registration Act in 1919 until 2019.

Useful websites

www.asanet.org/about/what-sociology

Watch sociologists explain what sociology is and their roles within it via a video on the American Sociological Association website. It provides a fascinating insight into what sociology can offer society.

www.nmc.org.uk/about-us/

Visit the NMC website to learn more about the role of the regulator concerning nursing standards and education.

www.britsoc.co.uk/what-is-sociology/

Learn more about sociology by visiting the British Sociological Association. You may find the information on their 'What is Sociology' page useful. It includes information on what sociologists do and related career pathways.

Chapter 2 Understanding individuals, their communities and wider society

Chapter aims

After reading this chapter, you will be able to:

- outline the contribution that nursing makes to individuals, communities and wider society;
- explain the social science ideas related to the individual, applying them to the role of nursing;
- discuss the concept of community inclusive of the strengths and assets that nurses can support people to draw upon;
- describe social science ideas related to society and relate these to contemporary nursing practice.

Introduction

This chapter will explore nursing practice from differing sociological and psychological perspectives. It explains how the social sciences provide a critical understanding of the role of professional practice at the level of individuals, communities and societies. Throughout the chapter, we will draw upon theoretical frameworks and research from sociology and psychology. This will help us explore how the social sciences relate to contemporary nursing practice.

Nursing's contribution

The nursing profession makes an important and varied contribution to the health of individuals, communities and wider society. We begin this chapter by briefly considering the broad scope of the nursing role. This understanding will be useful for later sections when considering how the social sciences support nurses in understanding people and their settings when providing care. The World Health Organization (WHO) (2019, page 1) explains that *nursing encompasses autonomous and collaborative care of individuals of all ages, families, groups and communities, sick or well and in all settings.* This definition shows why nurses must understand cultural, social and individual dynamics to meet people's care needs across diverse communities. They must be able to adjust their approaches to deliver personalised, effective treatment regardless of the patient's background, health condition or surroundings.

It is worth reflecting that the work of the nursing profession is situated in our increasingly globalised digital world. Digital and communications technology developments continue to further impact the provision of health and social care, including areas such as digital healthcare, big data and artificial intelligence. As shown in Figure 2.1, nurses and other healthcare practitioners can now consult with patients and colleagues regardless of distance, through the use of modern communications technology. They can also draw upon advanced diagnostic equipment and software to support clinical decision-making.

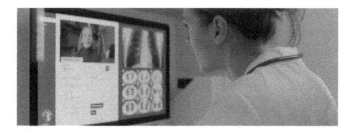

Figure 2.1   Delivering telemedicine to a patient

Source: supamotion – stock.adobe.com

These changes influence service delivery and how individuals receive healthcare information and treatment. Patients previously relied primarily on healthcare professionals for material and guidance about their conditions. Now individuals may conduct research into their health condition using online information that would not have been easily available to them in the past. On the other hand, service providers can use digital technology and large data sets to streamline and tailor their offerings. This can be useful when attempting to target specific at-risk communities. Nurses can use technology and scientific advances to support clinical care and assessment. Despite these developments, it is important to remember that caring remains at the centre of nursing work (Wall, 2010). They do not replace the importance of human interaction and should be used to enhance the capacity of nurses to deliver empathetic and patient-focused care.

Given the broad work of nurses and the increasingly interconnected world they operate within, it is worth keeping this in mind as we explore the social sciences in more detail. The following section will explore how the social sciences can assist nurses in developing understanding at the level of individuals, communities and broader society. There will be a focus on specific theoretical ideas relevant to the nursing profession and consideration of assets-based approaches.

Understanding the individual

Exploring different perspectives on what it means to be a person can help us to develop a richer understanding of the individual. We often think that we understand ourselves and that this helps us to understand others. While this may be true to an extent, it can also lead us to make assumptions about others. These judgements can become more pronounced when it comes to others from a different background to ours. Social science helps us establish a more objective understanding of individuals while considering contextual factors.

Sociological enquiry shows us that, in an increasingly individualised Western society, there has been a shift from group identity to individual identity. Globalisation has been one of the key drivers of this, requiring people to live in more open ways and respond to a changing interconnected world (Giddens and Sutton, 2021, page 145). This has been accompanied by a greater need for individuals to actively construct their identities, with less reliance on local group identities and influence through online environments. There has been a breaking down of some of the traditional social bonds, particularly in areas such as religion (Chase and Walker, 2013). It is now less common for large groups of extended families to live together. Individualistic understandings of modern life often focus on the behaviour and experiences of each person (Newman, 2014). These broadscale changes have been propagated by countless factors, including globalisation, technological developments, areas of increased social mobility (e.g. going to university) and in recent decades through the wide adoption of social media. Personal traits have become central to self-concept, favouring individual goals over group goals (Newman, 2014). Even in this context, the individual remains inseparable from our community and wider society, as we shall explore in later sections of this chapter.

Individualisation can be seen in nursing through an increased focus on care that is tailored to the specific preferences and needs of the person. Digital health technologies will only increase in the coming years, further enhancing individual choice and tailoring services. It brings forth a question: what does it mean to be an individual, and how can the social sciences help us to further unpick this concept?

Student voices: Tricia

You need to know how different people tick, and obviously it is exactly the same in nursing.

Tricia, 1st Year Adult Student Nurse

Activity 2.1   Reflection

Before starting her nurse education, Tricia (see the previous Student Voices box) had a job providing beauty treatments to clients. Have you ever been in a job or role at school/college where it was important to understand how people think and behave? Think about how these skills may transfer to your current nursing studies.

An outline answer is given at the end of the chapter.

At this point, it is helpful to consider psychological conceptions of what makes us human. In contrast with wider social inquiry, psychologists tend to focus more closely on the individual as their 'unit of analysis' when carrying out research. One broad area of interest is that of cognitive and biological psychology, exploring areas such as memory, cognition, temperament, anxiety and depression. Theoretical developments and the findings of psychological research can assist nurses and other healthcare professionals in better understanding the behaviour and needs of individuals, enabling them to provide tailored support or direct the person towards an appropriate service or agency. An example is the research that psychologists and others have undertaken into adverse childhood experiences, as discussed in the following Concept Summary on this topic.

Concept summary: Adverse childhood experiences

One area where a person's individual experiences can significantly impact their health outcomes is that of adverse childhood experiences (ACEs). ACEs may be defined as *highly stressful events or situations that happen during childhood and/or adolescence. It can be a single event, or prolonged threats to and/or breaches of a young person's safety, security, trust, or bodily integrity* (The British Psychological Association, 2019, page 1).

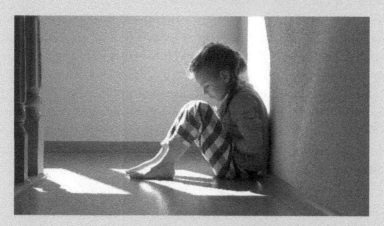

Figure 2.2   A child feels unsafe

Source: Erika Richard – stock.adobe.com

It may be challenging for nurses to understand and respond to the physical and mental effects that can be apparent in lifelong ways. Psychologists and other researchers are helping to show how these impacts affect a person's wellbeing and behaviour (Briggs et al., 2021; Brown et al., 2022; Seteanu and Giosan, 2021). Nurses, particularly those working in areas such as Health Visiting, play an important role in supporting families to reduce ACEs and prevent household adversity. People whose health and wellbeing are being affected by ACEs can be supported by nurses with the relevant training and competence or directed to specialist services. By engaging in training, reflective practice and peer support, you can become more aware of these issues and how to respond to them appropriately (Gilliver, 2018).

A theoretical perspective within psychology that has particular relevance to nursing is called humanistic psychology. The American psychologist Carl Rogers (1902–78) was influential in this field of enquiry. Rogers believed that rather than being shaped by external reality, our lives are actually shaped by our *perception* of external reality. He explains that we fundamentally live in a world of our own creation, and thus each person experiences the world in a way unique to them (Gross, 2020).

Concept summary: What is a theory?

A theory may be defined *as a set of ideas that claims to explain how something works* (Haralambos et al., 2013, page 9).

These ideas are central to Rogers' theoretical developments related to person-centred therapy. His work explains the role of empathy, unconditional positive regard and congruence within therapeutic relationships. Each of the three 'core conditions' refers to a specific quality that should be fostered to support an effective relationship. Empathy relates to a communicated understanding of the person's emotional and subjective perspective, unconditional positive regard refers to accepting and valuing the individual without judgement and congruence means genuineness, characterised by open and honest communication (Ruddick, 2010). Roger's work shows us that by being an attentive and careful listener while demonstrating acceptance and genuineness, we can facilitate relationships that are more likely to have a positive outcome (Dana and Upton, 2013). The influence of Roger's work can be found within current nursing approaches, such as person-centred care, where nurses should consider what makes each person unique and put their needs first (NMC, 2020a).

Activity 2.2 Reflection

Read the following article that will provide more information about person-centred care and its social science origins (ask your university library for assistance if you cannot access the article): Chapman, H (2017) Nursing theories 1: person-centred care. *Nursing Times* [online], 113(10): 59.

Consider two ways in which adopting a person-centred approach is important for your nursing practice.

An outline answer is provided at the end of the chapter.

Another influential theorist in the field of humanistic psychology is Abraham Maslow (1908–70). He developed the five-stage hierarchy of needs model, which is often displayed as a pyramid (see Figure 2.3). The pyramid is a representation of Maslow's

(1943) theory regarding the level of satisfaction a person might need to fulfil as they strive towards higher levels (Maslow, 1943). It helps to show how a person's basic needs must be met before they can move towards those further up the hierarchy. A person will be forced to prioritise their physiological needs if they do not have access to food, water or shelter. This is likely to compromise their ability to maintain other areas, such as personal security (i.e. they are likely to take greater risks to acquire things that are necessary for basic survival). However, the hierarchy is not strictly linear, and people may simultaneously be partially satisfied at different levels.

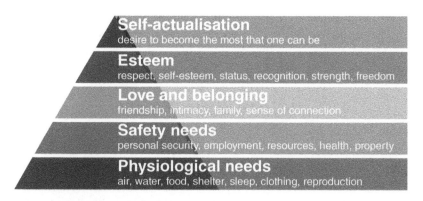

Figure 2.3 Maslow's hierarchy of needs

Source: laplateresca – stock.adobe.com

The hierarchy is relevant to nurses as it shows how supporting people with their needs can facilitate progress towards higher levels such as belonging, esteem and self-actualisation. The ideas from humanistic psychology lead us to the next section, which considers how nurses can use assets-based approaches to support individuals in meeting their unique needs.

Assets-based approaches at the individual level

Assets-based approaches require us to recognise the personal strengths and resources of each individual, exploring how they can use these to support health and wellbeing. Drawing on the ideas from humanistic psychology we considered earlier, person-centred conversations help us understand each person's strengths, preferences, aspirations and needs (National Institute for Clinical Excellence (NICE), 2019). A nurse can use communication skills to facilitate open discussions in which the person is encouraged to express their views, with input from carers, friends and family as appropriate. They need to display active listening skills so that the individual's assets, alongside any barriers, can be understood. This should establish positive areas of a person's life and support them to build upon these while accounting for the health outcomes that they care about. The person's independence should be promoted as far as possible, including the promotion of positive risk-taking (NICE, 2019). Achieving a balance between safety and autonomy can contribute to improved self-esteem, resilience and overall quality of life for the individual, fostering their sense of control and dignity.

The following is a case study example showing the positive outcome that an asset-based approach can have. It is related to a Family Nurse Partnership (FNP), an evidence-based programme that provides support for first-time mothers under the age of 20 (Scottish Government, 2020). The programme involves a structured home visiting programme that specially trained nurses deliver from pregnancy through to the child's second birthday. The nurse uses approaches designed to support positive relationships and caregiving, promote health behaviour change and increase access to additional services within the local community. The case study is a shortened version of an evaluation report into FNPs by the Scottish Government (2019a, page 44).

Case study: Family Nurse Partnerships

Jodie enrolled in the programme aged 15, when she was 12 weeks pregnant. She had previously experienced a range of adverse experiences including physical abuse, sexual abuse, unstable housing and a period of homelessness. Jodie was attending Child and Adolescent Mental Health Services (CAMHS) to deal with self-harm and emotional difficulties. Jodie lived with her partner's family and was thought to have made good preparations for her baby, helped by her partner's mum. Her father provided financial support. Jodie engaged well during her pregnancy with FNP, CAMHS and her midwife, forming a good therapeutic and trusting relationship with her Family Nurse. At birth, Jodie's baby was placed on the Child Protection Register but was removed after three months because of the positive nature of relationship between Jodie and her baby. Social Work planned to remain involved on a voluntary basis. Although painful, Jodie broke off her relationship with her own mother because of her concerns of risks of harm from her mother's alcoholism to her baby. Jodie is reported as having made good progress during her engagement with the programme, in particular by managing the stressors that affected her mood and by learning how to meet all of her baby's physical and emotional needs. She often phoned or texted her Family Nurse with any worries or anxieties regarding her or her baby's health and well-being. Jodie re-engaged with education and completed her fourth year at school, securing a place at college to study childcare.

Through the assets-based approach evident within the scenario, the FNP plays an important role in breaking down intergenerational cycles of neglect and child maltreatment (Scottish Government, 2019a). During the COVID-19 pandemic, the FNP moved to an online/video consulting service to ensure continued delivery. Telehealth interventions were introduced, with around half of the visits completed this way (Scottish Government, 2021).

An evaluation of the FNP and full case study are linked in the Further Reading section of this chapter.

When supporting a person with their health needs, it is often useful to share information with the person about resources and support within the local community, including peer support services. Where appropriate, consult a practitioner who knows about local services, including those provided by the voluntary and community sector (NICE, 2019). Nurses should also explore potential barriers, such as transport and language, identifying sources of support for the individual. A related area is health literacy, which involves a person's ability to understand and use health information (NHS, 2021). This is a significant issue, with a study by Rowlands et al. (2015) finding that 43 per cent of participants had literacy skills below the level required to understand health materials fully. To learn more, you can access a health literacy toolkit developed by NHS Health Education England (2023), designed specifically for health and social care workers. The toolkit contains useful information and resources; you can find it in the Useful Websites section at the end of this chapter.

Earlier, we briefly considered the proliferation of digital technologies and their relevance to the work of nurses. When supporting a person, establishing if they have access to digital resources is essential. There may be potential barriers, such as digital poverty, where a person has poor access to technology and high speed internet, perhaps due to a lack of broadband or the required equipment. Additionally, they may have difficulties and a lack of confidence when engaging with health services and information in a digital format. There are organisations and services that you may be able to direct the person towards so that they can gain support with issues relating to the use of technology.

An example is the Digital Poverty Alliance (2022), which is developing a directory of support agencies and services. It is also worth being aware of NHS (2019b) guidance promoting digital inclusion within health and social care. Links to both these sources of information and support relating to digital poverty can be found in this chapter's Further Reading section.

Understanding communities

When people think of nursing it often revolves around the image of a nurse working in a hospital setting, an impression largely shaped by personal experiences, hospital visits or television dramas like *Casualty*. In these hospital settings, nurses must understand the cultural and social aspects of the local communities that their patients call home. This knowledge not only helps them guide patients on how to manage their conditions after discharge but also helps them tap into local resources.

However, a large proportion of nursing takes place beyond hospital walls and into the heart of local communities. Nurses work in a variety of roles in community settings, including Health Visitors, Community Mental Health Nurses, Community Nurses and District Nurses. These positions give them invaluable insights into community members' living conditions and lifestyles, shaping their understanding of effectively supporting their health and wellbeing. The word 'community' will be one that you frequently encounter during your nursing studies and while on placement. Which leads us to ask the question: what is a community?

As with many apparently simple concepts, the answer is complex. As a sociological concept, 'community' has fallen in and out of favour over the years. This is partly due to difficulties in establishing what a community is and how to study it. A traditional human community might be defined as a group of people who live together within a defined physical and social space. However, this type of definition does not fully address modern conceptions of community in our digital and globalised world. There now tends to be less focus on physical space than in the past, with many people interacting in diverse online communities.

As a student nurse, understanding the fabric of the communities you serve is important to help recognise the complex interconnections between individuals. These connections span diverse aspects such as gender relations, work dynamics, unemployment, housing, ethnicity and migration patterns (Crow, 2014). Structural inequalities often underscore these communities, making some more susceptible to issues like unemployment (Scottish Government, 2019b). Inequalities will be explored further in Chapter 4. Regardless of the issues different communities face, understanding those we work with helps us identify the challenges and opportunities within them. Using this knowledge, nurses can collaborate with community networks, support groups and third-sector organisations to improve people's health and wellbeing. This approach can make a real difference in people's lives by addressing their needs in a more nuanced and comprehensive manner.

From a psychological perspective, a community can imbue feelings of belonging and emotional connection, often built upon shared experiences, history and identity (Brodsky and Marx, 2001). Community-based services enable people to live within their community rather than having to live within an institutional setting, as was often the case in the past. These services include day centres, supported housing and outreach

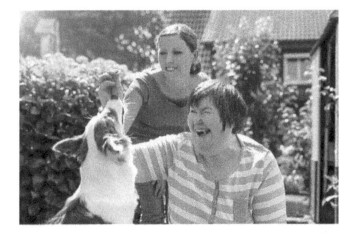

Figure 2.4   A person receives community-based care

Source: M.Dörr and M.Frommherz – stock.adobe.com

provisions. They benefit people by enabling them to live without the constraints of institutional care. This extends to simple things such as being able to keep a pet dog (as shown in Figure 2.4), an unlikely option within formal settings.

Concept summary: Dementia Friendly Communities

During your nurse education, it is likely that you will encounter people with dementia. Dementia Friendly Communities can support the psychological needs of people with dementia (Lin, 2017). They can be defined as follows:

A Dementia Friendly Community can involve a wide range of people, organisations, and geographical areas. A DFC recognises that a person with dementia is more than their diagnosis, and that everyone has a role to play in supporting their independence and inclusion.

(Buckner et al., 2019, page 1235)

Community assets create 'social capital', resources such as support, volunteering networks and links which help to empower people while bridging divides of access and knowledge (Rippon and Hopkins, 2015). People with dementia need access to local networks, contributing to a sense of belonging that is part of the glue that binds people and places together (Rahman and Swaffer, 2018). Nurses play a key role in supporting people with dementia to be as independent and included as possible.

Community strengths and assets

Assets-based health approaches have a different starting point from traditional health and social care services. They are founded upon the question 'What makes us healthy?' instead of the deficit-based question 'What makes us ill?' (Rippon and Hopkins, 2015, page 3). This means that services should move away from 'doing things to' communities or deficit-based approaches and towards 'doing things with' communities or assets-based approaches. Materially deprived communities may be rich in community relations, resources and creativity (Friedli, 2013). The most frequently cited definition of a 'health asset' is the following:

any factor (or resource), which enhances the ability of individuals, groups, communities, populations, social systems and /or institutions to maintain and sustain health and well-being and to help to reduce health inequities. These assets can operate at the level of the individual, group, community, and /or population 'as protective (or promoting) factors to buffer against life's stresses.

(Morgan and Ziglio, 2007, page 18)

This approach aims to improve the wellbeing of all community members, rather than campaigns and services designed to change community behaviour according to service priorities and targets. Traditional public health models remain important but should be complemented by approaches that capitalise upon community assets (Van Bortel et al., 2019). It is about building community assets and strengths by engaging with and empowering members of the community, thus promoting participation and partnership.

Concept summary: The salutogenic model of health

A theory related to the concept of asset-based approaches is the Israeli American sociologist Antonovsky's salutogenic model of health. Salutogenesis means the 'origins of health', *genesis* means 'origins' and *saluto* means 'health', which moves the focus away from disease towards supporting health and wellbeing (Vinje et al., 2017). Antonovsky's salutogenic model of health was devised as a resource-oriented concept, focusing specifically on stress management. He aimed to understand why some people maintain their health even in stressful situations and use these health-promoting factors to boost resilience (Pérez-Wilson et al., 2020). The salutogenic model is useful in showing the active and dynamic process of maintaining health in the face of life's unavoidable stressors. The model emphasises how we constantly interact with and adapt to stressors in order to maintain our wellbeing.

One of your responsibilities as a nurse is to assist people in identifying and utilising community resources and assets (NHS Greater Glasgow and Clyde, 2017). As your career progresses, focusing on developing networks and relationships within the local community is essential. This will help to give you a thorough understanding of local resources, which you can use to help people with their health (NICE, 2019). You should always respect and draw upon the knowledge, skills and connections of individuals who are members of the community. By doing so, you can capitalise on and promote the development of the community's existing assets and strengths.

Activity 2.3   Critical thinking

Undertake an internet search to find three health assets in your local area that may support people with a long-term health condition. You might choose a condition related to diabetes, mental health issues, heart problems, strokes or respiratory problems.

Begin by searching for local charities and community groups related to your topic that may be available locally, then look through their website to see what resources and support they offer. Next, check the NHS website for your area to see if they highlight any community groups or resources that may be available.

Finally, think about how easy or difficult it was to find information about health assets within the community. Can you identify any ways in which access to the information could be improved for those with a long-term condition?

An outline answer is given at the end of the chapter.

Connections between people within communities provide a source of resilience, support and control, supporting their health and wellbeing. Nurses and other professionals should adopt a partnership approach that values collaboration with the community and cultivates integration across services (Marshall and Easton, 2018). This will help promote the assets that contribute to good health within the community while fostering local networks that support community cohesion. Reducing preventable health inequalities, which are sometimes referred to as health inequities, among the community is a core aim of the approach. We'll explore these in more detail within Chapter 4.

Communities of practice

One aspect of nursing is that you will often work as part of a group with other health and social care professionals working towards the same goals. In a sense, this is itself a community through its shared values, practices and customs. Communities of Practice is a social learning theory originally proposed by Lave and Wenger (1991) and then further developed by Wenger (1998). This theory is especially relevant to nursing because it illuminates the type of learning you will experience during your placements. It explains learning as *situated*, which means that it occurs through participation within a community of practice (Lave and Wenger, 1991). In the context of your nursing education, you will most likely be a member of two communities of practice simultaneously. One community is your university, where you interact with other students and your lecturers, sharing knowledge and experiences. The other community you will encounter is within your clinical placement setting, where you will interact with professionals, patients and other stakeholders while gaining practical experience and real-world insights. Participating in both communities allows you to combine theoretical knowledge with practical application, enhancing your learning experience.

The term 'legitimate peripheral participation' is important in placement experiences. It refers to the transition of newcomers towards becoming full members of a community of practice (Lave and Wenger, 1991). The term 'legitimate' refers to the learner's acceptance or recognition as a potential member of the community. The term 'peripheral' implies that the newcomer begins their education on the outskirts or periphery of the community. 'Participation' refers to active involvement in social community practices and the construction of identities in relation to these communities. As a result, the term implies that learning occurs through gradually increasing participation in a community, moving from the periphery (where the newcomer observes and learns from more experienced members) to the centre as they gain expertise. It should be noted that full status may not be fully attained during shorter placements.

The social structures of the community, including roles such as Practice Assessor and Practice Supervisor, can help a newcomer progress towards deeper involvement. This process can either empower or push a newcomer to the margins, depending on how much support and guidance they receive to engage at the appropriate level. Participating in a community of practice as a nursing student during your placement and your placement will open the door to enriching learning opportunities (Grealish and Ranse, 2009). Non-participation due to marginalisation, on the other hand, can impede learning and potentially have a negative impact on your emerging identity as a nurse (Molesworth, 2017). Read the case study featuring Bernadette and Abigail to apply this theory to common circumstances that arise during nursing students' placements.

Case study: Bernadette and Abigail

Remember Bernadette and Abigail from Chapter 1? These were the two student nurses who started their education at the same time and have become friends. Bernadette is in placement on an orthopaedic (specialising in the skeletal system) ward, where the staff are very welcoming. She met her Practice Assessor and Practice Supervisors on day one and regularly practises alongside them. Whenever an interesting procedure or intervention occurs, the Practice Supervisor ensures Bernadette can be involved to help her meet her learning objectives. Over time this has helped her get to know more of the staff, and she is getting more knowledgeable about how the team works together. Meanwhile, Abigail also has a placement in another orthopaedic ward at the same hospital. The placement area is having staffing issues, and Abigail did not meet her Practice Assessor and Practice Supervisor until the week after she started. Although the ward has been friendly, she has felt a bit lost during the placement. Arrangements for her to work with someone from the team always seem a bit last minute. On several occasions, they have asked her just to be available to help as required. Although she was busy during these shifts, there was little structure, and she made limited progress with her learning objectives. Abigail has become aware of interesting procedures and interventions after they have taken place without her involvement, and the staff always apologise and mention how busy it has been.

Activity 2.4 Reflection

From the perspective of communities of practice can you recognise any aspect of participation and marginalisation within the case study?

What might Abigail do to address the situation?

An outline answer is given at the end of the chapter.

Understanding society

When you consider the term 'society', what comes to mind? It may bring forth ideas of how human life is organised. These may stem from the society where you grew up or live today. When many people come together in a sustained manner, sharing factors such as place and culture, this can be thought of as a society. Collective social interconnection and the development of institutions provide broad structures within which life is organised. Within a particular context, people adapt to their environment and each other. This process means that, in a sense, the individual retreats as they conform to the shared norms associated with living within a specific social and cultural arena.

Concept summary: Norms

A norm is a sociological concept that describes the rules of behaviour that reflect or embody a culture's values, either prescribing a given type of behaviour or forbidding it (Giddens and Sutton, 2021, page 966).

With their focus on human behaviour, psychologists sometimes explore behaviour at the societal level. One interesting area where this came into prominence was during the response to COVID-19. Here psychologists, with their interest in human behaviour, played a significant role in many governments' responses to the pandemic. They advised on how to ensure the population displayed the desired behaviours in response to the public health crisis. This is something we will explore in more detail within Chapter 6. Despite the perspectives put forward in psychology, the study of society is primarily the domain of sociology. Indeed, sociology is often described as 'the study of society'.

Nursing practice takes place within these structures of society, so we need to explore the work of the sociologists who have studied it. The first thing to mention is that there are different ways in which society can be viewed and understood. Indeed, there is no universally agreed way to analyse and interpret our complex human societies. There is a debate within sociology as to whether society, in the industrial, democratic and national sense, should remain the core level of sociological analysis given globalisation and the digital revolution discussed earlier (Dubet, 2021). Society is not static. It changes over time and place, even if some of the institutions persist. For example, think back over recent decades to consider how the digital revolution has changed how we bank, shop and communicate with one another (complete Activity 2.4 to think more deeply about this topic).

People and institutions attempt to adapt as new technological innovations have become available. This constant adaptation represents our ability to learn, innovate and progress as we shape and are shaped by the changing society around us. A key sociological concept that helps us understand the relationship between the individual and wider society is that of the sociological imagination (see Concept Summary: The Sociological Imagination). As a student nurse, the development of a sociological imagination is one way to better grasp individual health and wellbeing, not just in terms of personal circumstances but also in the context of broader societal influences. It will help you to link personal experiences and behaviours to societal patterns and trends.

Concept summary: The sociological imagination

The sociological imagination is a concept originally established by the American sociologist known as C Wright Mills (1916–62). It invites us to address the complex relationship between a person and the social world around them (Murji et al., 2022). Applying the sociological imagination helps us recognise and make sense of how personal problems become wider societal issues. It also encourages us to apply a critical lens to how society may create the conditions for these individual problems and prevent the person from escaping them. C Wright Mills' 1959 text of the same name explores these issues and, despite their age, the principles behind the concept remain of relevance today. As nurses, we often encounter people who are experiencing hardships in their life. Developing an ability to recognise how these play into wider social issues that require attention is important. A nurse who can recognise how the conditions of a person's life may be influencing their present problems has a broader outlook and is thus in a better position to adopt an empathetic approach while avoiding inappropriate blame.

Activity 2.5   Reflection

Today's world is more connected than ever; people can collaborate, share ideas and instantly communicate over long distances. Go back a few decades and the situation was very different, with digital technologies still in their infancy.

To learn more about the impact of these changes, speak to an older adult about the digital advances that have occurred during their lives. Ask them about the most significant technological changes they've witnessed and how they felt about these changes. Contrast these with your thoughts and experiences.

An outline answer is given at the end of the chapter.

There are several classical perspectives on society, each presenting contrasting views. We'll briefly look at two of these: functionalism and conflict theory. They are referred to as structural theories because they put forward ideas about how and why society is structured the way it is. Sociological enquiry has developed and diverged from these original ideas as time has passed and the discipline has developed. Nonetheless, it is useful to understand these core frameworks within sociology as they provide background to contemporary sociological enquiry applied to nursing throughout the book.

Functionalism is a paradigm that suggests society is made up of interconnected parts that provide stability by working together. An analogy commonly used when people are first learning about functionalism is to compare the understanding of society with that of the human body. This seems fitting because we are nurses and familiar with the human body. Each body system plays a vital role in the health of the person. If there is a problem with the cardiovascular system, it can affect other systems and threaten the person's overall health. Similarly, a stable society requires that all the 'systems', or institutions, operate effectively. These institutions usually include those such as education, health, policing and justice, and local government. From a nursing perspective, we can understand nursing and healthcare provision more widely as, in simple terms, a fundamental part of a consensus-based system that helps society function correctly.

Conflict theory also recognises the importance of social structures within society. In contrast with functionalism. This perspective rejects the idea that these structures are benign and work towards a common goal. Instead, it highlights the competitive struggle across and within the structures and groups in society and the inequalities and power issues arising from the resultant divisions (Giddens and Sutton, 2021). Karl Marx was an influential proponent of these issues, exposing the ways society is structured according to the values and needs of the economic structure of society (Punch et al., 2013). From a nursing perspective, we might take a critical view of nursing and the medical profession, considering how it maintains the workforce/consumer to benefit the economic system. Another conflict theory is that of feminism. This has relevance for the nursing profession and is an area we will explore more deeply within Chapter 5.

Scenario: Sofia

Imagine you are a student nurse working with the Community Mental Health Service in Scotland. You are caring for a 34-year-old woman called Sofia. She is a person who uses drugs and has been displaying symptoms of depression over the past year. Sofia has an infected sore on her leg that requires regular dressing but is beginning to heal. Unfortunately, Sofia recently received a letter from her landlord informing her that the property containing her flat is being sold. She does not have alternative accommodation and is worried she may become homeless. While providing care to Sofia, your Practice

(Continued)

Supervisor encourages you to think about the potential health impact of her housing circumstances. You remember learning about the sociological imagination and how the concept may help to analyse the connection between wider social influences and individual experience.

Activity 2.6   Critical thinking

Using your sociological imagination, explain the relationship between societal issues and Sofia's personal circumstances.

An outline answer is given at the end of the chapter.

Chapter summary

During this chapter, we have seen the contribution that nursing makes to individuals, communities and wider society. As a person on a journey towards becoming a registered nurse, you may have identified ways that the social sciences relate to your current and future experiences. This might concern how assets-based approaches can promote health and wellbeing for individuals and communities or how social science theory and research can help you understand the context of nursing work. We hope you also better grasp key concepts such as society and its interdependent relationship with individuals and their communities. In the next chapter, we will build upon how you can understand the social sciences to help meet people's unique holistic care needs.

Activities: Brief outline answers

Activity 2.1   Reflection

Tricia felt her prior experiences of working with people were beneficial for understanding the individual within nursing. Were you able to relate to her points? Often roles that involve dealing with others while providing services and problem-solving help us to develop our communication skills. These transfer to nursing, where effective communication is essential to person-centred care.

Activity 2.2   Reflection

What are two ways in which adopting a person-centred approach is important for your nursing practice?

After reading the article by Chapman (2017) you may have identified that this approach will support partnership working with service users, promoting their self-esteem and self-efficacy.

Activity 2.3　Critical thinking

Undertake an internet search to find three health assets in your local area that may support people with a long-term health condition.

Following your search, you likely will have found that the major health conditions have charitable organisations and support groups with resources available within your area. If there were no local assets, expand your search to include the wider country within which you live. Less common conditions may have limited resources available, but hopefully, you found some related support. The NHS may also have provided some useful information and links. Improving access to information is important – perhaps things like a repository of support services in your area would be useful if this does not currently exist.

Activity 2.4　Reflection

You may have found that there were aspects of marginalisation within Abigail's situation. Meanwhile, Bernadette is experiencing greater participation within the community of practice. Abigail should consider explaining how she feels to the placement area and ask them to agree a plan to enable her to progress further towards her learning objective. She should also contact her tutor from the university for support. There may be guidance within her practice learning documentation that she can follow. Abigail would benefit from doing this during the earlier stages of the placement rather than putting it off. She should also engage in the placement evaluation process to help ensure other students do not have the same experiences.

Activity 2.5　Reflection

When speaking with an older adult, you may have found that the use of technology has increased substantially over the years. It will hopefully have been interesting hearing how these changes have impacted life, perhaps with consideration of the pros and cons of the changes. After you've heard their stories, think about your own.

- How have technological advancements influenced your life?
- How do your reactions to these developments differ from theirs?

Understanding the differences and similarities in your experiences might help you better understand how technology impacts people at different stages of life.

Activity 2.6　Critical thinking

You may have considered how culture, politics and economics influence individual behaviour. Issues such as poverty, unemployment, education and social isolation can all impact drug use, while stigmatisation can prevent people like Sofia from getting the support they need. You may also have considered how homelessness is a societal issue as well as a personal one. It is linked to larger social issues, such as unemployment, a lack of affordable housing and a lack of support for people facing financial difficulties. Sofia's situation also impacts society. As the number of people facing similar difficulties rises, this is likely to affect wider societal structures and culture.

Further reading

Scottish Government (2019) Family Nurse Partnership in Scotland: Revaluation report.

You can review an evaluation of the FNP and the full case discussed in 'Case study: Family Nurse Partnerships'. The report can be accessed at: www.gov.scot/publications/revaluation-family-nurse-partnership-scotland/ (Accessed: 27 June 2023).

Giddens, A and Sutton, PW (2021) *Sociology*. Cambridge: Polity.

For a detailed examination of the sociological issues explored in this chapter, and many others, it is worth accessing a foundational textbook for sociology. You will find there are many options to buy or loan via any university library. Sociology is one such useful text and we refer to this book several times within this chapter.

Gross, R (2020) *Psychology: The science of mind and behaviour*. 8th ed. London: Hodder Education.

For a detailed examination of the psychological issues explored in this chapter, and many others, it is worth accessing a foundational textbook on psychology. You will find there are many options to buy or loan via any university library. A useful text is *Psychology*. This is another book we have referred to several times within this chapter.

Rippon, S and Hopkins, T (2015) Head, hands and heart: Asset-based approaches in health care. The Health Foundation.

Read 'Head, Hands and Heart' to learn more about asset-based approaches within healthcare The article can be accessed at: www.health.org.uk/publications/head-hands-and-heart-asset-based-approaches-in-health-care (Accessed: 27 June 2023).

NHS Digital (2019) Digital inclusion guide for health and social care, NHS choices.

Learn how the NHS (2019b) is promoting digital inclusion by reading through the information on their website. The guide is available at: https://digital.nhs.uk/about-nhs-digital/corporate-information-and-documents/digital-inclusion (Accessed: 27 June 2023).

Useful websites

www.nmc.org.uk/standards/code/code-in-action/person-centred-care/

Watch this short video by the NMC on person-centred care. While watching, think about how you might apply this in your next placement.

https://digitalpovertyalliance.org/dpa-directory-for-support/

Find out more information about the support available for digital poverty by visiting the Digital Poverty Alliance directory of services.

https://cms.bps.org.uk/sites/default/files/2022-06/Briefing%20Paper%20-%20Adverse%20 Childhood%20Experiences_0.pdf

Learn more about ACEs by reading information available from the British Psychological Society.

https://library.nhs.uk/wp-content/uploads/sites/4/2023/06/Health-Literacy-Toolkit.pdf

This is the second edition of the Health Literacy Toolkit published by NHS Health Education England (2023). The resources contains useful information and resources for health and social care workers.

Chapter 3　Holistic care

Introduction

This chapter considers how the social sciences enable nurses to account for the holistic care needs of their patients. It will help you recognise how they underpin fundamental approaches within nursing practice, including empathetic and patient-centred care. Reflecting upon the development of the biopsychosocial model will show how a complete approach to nursing care can provide benefits over those which are more one-dimensional. Within this chapter, we will also explore how holistic care can support care planning and provide opportunities to recognise the lived experience of those receiving care.

What is holistic care?

Holistic care means providing care beyond focusing on a person's medical needs, enabling the nursing team to support their wider needs. This approach is why proponents of holistic care emphasise the importance of looking beyond scientific, materialistic medicine towards a broader recognition of mind, body and spirit (Dossey and Dossey, 1998). Despite the popularity of the term 'holistic care' within the nursing literature, it does not have a universally accepted definition. There is, however, a consensus that it involves *whole person care* (Frisch and Rabinowitsch, 2019, page 262). Holistic care involves taking into account factors such as the person's social, physical, psychological, spiritual, cultural and emotional needs. Rather than focusing on a person's specific health conditions, this approach means the wider needs of the individual are recognised. It can present opportunities to enhance the person's overall health and wellbeing, improving outcomes and reducing the likelihood of recurring problems.

Scenario: Carolina

Imagine you are working in a nursing home. Your Practice Supervisor asks you to be involved in care planning for one of the patients with dementia. The patient, Carolina, is a 70-year-old lady who was diagnosed with dementia one year previously. She could not care for herself at home and was admitted approximately six months ago. You started the placement four weeks ago and have enjoyed getting to know the residents. Carolina enjoys reminiscing. Due to her condition, she becomes easily confused and gets very anxious in unfamiliar situations. She likes singing, and the home has recently introduced a sing-along session with a local professional singer. During discussions with Carolina and her family, it was agreed that she would benefit from attending.

Activity 3.1   Decision-making

- Identify two of Carolina's holistic care needs.
- Think of two approaches that may reduce the likelihood of Carolina becoming anxious when joining the sing-along session.

An outline answer is given at the end of the chapter.

When the NHS was founded in 1948, its founding principles were to meet everyone's needs, to be free at the point of delivery and to be based on clinical needs rather than financial ability. However, the care practice at the time was more medically oriented, primarily focusing on disease diagnosis and treatment. The patient was regarded as a 'case' of a particular disease rather than as a whole person. Patients' mental, emotional and social needs were generally regarded as secondary, if at all. In the 1960s and 1970s, healthcare began to shift towards a more patient-centred approach. This was influenced by a variety of social changes, as well as the introduction of new medical technologies and medicines. With the rise of holistic and integrative medicine in the 1980s and 1990s, there was a growing recognition of the need to see the patient as a whole person. This included the biopsychosocial model of care, which you will read about later in the chapter. Healthcare professionals began to recognise that physical health could not be separated from mental health and that a person's social environment significantly impacted their health.

The concept of holistic care has become even more deeply embedded in the NHS in recent years. The rising prevalence of chronic diseases and an ageing population have necessitated a more comprehensive, patient-centred approach. The NHS (2019a) Long Term Plan includes measures which promote holistic care, including a greater emphasis on prevention, individualised care and mental health. It's worth noting that while the NHS has made significant progress towards holistic care, obstacles still exist. There are resource constraints, staff shortages and systemic issues to consider. You may find you have an important role in advocating for and implementing holistic care during your placements.

Why is holistic care important?

Holistic care is important for many reasons, so let us consider three important examples. Firstly, it helps promote the overall health and wellbeing of the person. Medical needs rarely occur in isolation, with most health issues impacting our wider life and vice versa. For example, most of us have experienced the flu: think about the effect on your life if you need to stay in bed for a couple of days. Try Activity 3.2 to think more deeply about your holistic care needs. Secondly, it can help address the root causes of any immediate health concerns. If we only treat the medical issue without accounting for the person's wider needs, then there is more chance it will worsen or recur. Imagine a person receiving treatment for an injured leg after a fall at home. A holistic approach may assist with identifying and supporting the person to reduce the risk of another fall when they return home. Thirdly, it recognises the person as a unique individual with a lived history. This approach is closely aligned with the NMC (2018c) *Code of professional standards*, and we'll consider lived experience later in this chapter.

Activity 3.2 Reflection

Think about a time that you were admitted to hospital for over a week. If you haven't experienced this, try to imagine that you require an extended stay in hospital for treatment. Think about your holistic care needs. Write down one factor or need that the nurses caring for you may benefit from being aware of:

1. Social
2. Physical
3. Emotional
4. Psychological
5. Spiritual
6. Cultural
7. Environmental

An outline answer is given at the end of the chapter.

Holistic care can help avoid poor practices such as overly routinised care that does not account for the individual's needs. It can help prevent the person being viewed through the prism of their immediate health condition, evident in approaches such as calling someone by their condition rather than name: *the diabetic in bed one*, for example. Although this was common in the past, it represents a form of dehumanisation that can contribute to a culture of care which is not individualised and may lead to poor care. A well-known example of poor care can be found in the Francis Report (UK Government, 2013). It was a seminal investigation into the Mid Staffordshire

NHS Foundation Trust's failings between 2005 and 2009. The report demonstrated the dire consequences of substandard care. Its findings show that institutionalised forms of care can harm patients (see Concept Summary: Institutionalised Care). The inquiry found the services provided by Mid Staffordshire NHS Foundation Trust lacked patient care, compassion, dignity and respect. It shared evidence of patients being neglected, starved and in pain. This was not merely a failure of individual practitioners but resulted from a system-wide culture of neglect and poor standards of care that became institutionalised. The failings were exacerbated by poor leadership and governance within the trust. The report showed how a culture prioritising targets and finances over patient welfare eroded nursing values. It reminded all of us in the nursing profession that we must prioritise patient comfort, safety and wellbeing. It also highlighted the importance of being able to speak up about patient safety concerns without fear of repercussions.

Given all the benefits of holistic care and the risks associated with institutionalised care, it will not come as a surprise that there continues to be a call for greater consideration of the social, relational and psychological aspects of a person's needs (Corral-Liria et al., 2022). Care needs to be tailored to the specific environment in which you provide care. The provision of holistic care is likely to be different if you work in an operating theatre instead of a long-term nursing home. Regardless of the setting, respecting each person and their unique needs remains important. The discussion will now consider the theoretical basis for approaches supporting this type of care.

Concept summary: Institutionalised care

Institutionalised care describes a way of providing health and social care services in a manner that prioritises the needs of the service over the needs of the individual. It was evident in modes of care that were highly structured and routinised. Within this framework, individual choice was often restricted. It could be argued that this presented a form of dehumanisation in the more extreme cases, presenting fertile ground for abuse.

Further information regarding institutionalised care and how to prevent it can be found in a short overview from the Social Care Institute for Excellence in *Commissioning care homes: common safeguarding challenges* – more details can be found in the Further Reading section of this chapter.

There have been large shifts away from this type of care, with many social care institutions being changed or closed down in the latter part of the last century. At the same time, there has been an increased focus on 'person-centred care', as discussed in Chapter 2. However, vigilance is required to ensure that there is no return towards institutionalised modes of care (Goodman, 2013).

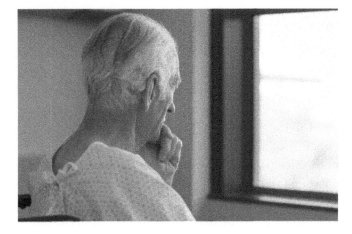

Figure 3.1   A concerned man looks out of the window

Source: iStock.com/Ridofranz

Holistic care is supported through a broad grasp of the different theoretical perspectives that inform nursing practice. These include the social science disciplines alongside others, including anatomy and physiology. We can see this recognised by a student nurse participating in research by Mowforth, Harrison and Morris (2005, page 45). When reflecting on their studies, the student highlighted how these disciplines come together to support holistic care: *it paints a wider picture, so you are not fixing on one aspect. You are actually looking for causes from psychology to sociology to link up the biology.* These disciplines are insufficient to fully account for holistic care, as this would negate aspects such as spirituality and cultural care, but they provide a good starting point.

The biopsychosocial approach

The biopsychosocial model acknowledges and attempts to address health's biological, psychological and social components. The biopsychosocial model of health came about partly in response to growing discontent with what is referred to as the medical model of health. The medical model of health emphasises and prioritises the physical aspect of ill health, often drawing criticism for disregarding the person and their wider needs. During the 1970s, some prominent thinkers deeply criticised Western approaches to healthcare. They pointed out the potential harms that healthcare and the drug industry can present. For example, Engel (1977) psychiatry argued for a move away from exclusive reliance on the biomedical model within psychiatric care. These debates continue today, as can be seen in the debate regarding the way some medications have the potential to lead to addiction and problems for the individual and society. Issues such as these are sometimes referred to as iatrogenesis, which is defined in the Concept Summary: Iatrogenesis.

> ## Concept summary: Iatrogenesis
>
> Iatrogenesis may be defined as harm caused by healthcare and medical interventions.

The biopsychosocial model has been positively evaluated and embraced in several areas of healthcare, although there is a lack of awareness of the approach more broadly (Wade and Halligan, 2017). The harm may arise from errors, such as misdiagnosis, but can also occur in the absence of any mistake. One such area is the application of the model during different stages of the lifespan. For example, Van Rickstal et al. (2022) show the interconnectedness of physical, social and mental wellbeing when considering the needs and preferences of those requiring end-of-life care. Additionally, specific areas of healthcare have embraced this approach more than others: an example is the biopsychosocial model of lower back pain. In support of this, Kamper et al. (2015) showed that a co-ordinated intervention for chronic lower back pain, incorporating the domains of the biopsychosocial model, can provide improvements over the standard care approaches. Now that we have considered the biopsychosocial approach let's return to the broader concept of holistic care and its relationship with the social sciences.

How social science informs holistic care

Sociology has an important role in the development of holistic practice. This was apparent within Aranda and Law's (2007, page 563) analysis of the views of student nurses and lecturers on the role of sociology in nursing. They described how understanding sociology led to *better holistic care during practice*. This included how sociology improved understanding of patients' *cultural influences and background* and supported holistic care planning. Psychology can also inform holistic care, by providing insights into the individual's psychological, cognitive and emotional needs.

Holistic care planning

To promote holistic approaches, the management of a patient's care plan should incorporate biological, psychological, social and spiritual aspects (Boswell et al., 2013, page 330). It is essential to seek meanings associated with the patient's experience, going beyond superficiality to *search for the roots* and improve understanding (Corral-Liria et al., 2022). Henry et al. (2014) emphasise that a holistic assessment is concerned with the whole person and involves gathering information to develop an understanding of their needs. This assists with tailoring care more effectively and can promote self-care due to the enhanced support and guidance that can follow. A holistic needs assessment may take time and patience, and care is required to avoid overburdening the person (Sandsund et al., 2020). It can be beneficial in a range of settings, from inpatients with cancer (Henry et al., 2014) to those accessing primary care for advance care planning due to the advancement of dementia (Tilburgs et al., 2018). As well as care planning, holistic care can also support discharge planning. A study by Mowforth, Harrison and Morris (2005, page 45), one student nurse links experiences of discharge planning to sociology:

> *When I studied sociology, I could not see the relevance at all … suddenly when I was doing discharge planning everything seemed to come together and I could see why it was so important.*

The delivery of holistic care can improve recovery and reduce hospital stays (Jasemi et al., 2017). This means there are improved outcomes for the patient and has been shown to reduce readmission rates (Fadol et al., 2019). A person who receives surgery in hospital following a fall at home for a fracture to their leg may be at risk of a similar problem reoccurring if they are discharged without any further assessment or support, for example. A better outcome is likely if the person's home circumstances and ability to manage are accounted for within their overall care.

Scenario: Austin

Imagine that you are working in a community hospital on a ward which specialises in stroke rehabilitation. You are caring for a 58-year-old man called Austin. He had a stroke one month ago, leaving him with left-sided weakness and problems with speech. His ability to mobilise has been improving; he can now mobilise with a standing aid and the assistance of one nurse. Austin has recently been moved from a soft diet to a normal diet with input from the dietician. Due to reduced strength and dexterity in his arm, he requires meals cut up and uses a plate with high rims. You are working with your Practice Supervisor to plan for Austin's discharge. He feels anxious about leaving the community hospital and worries about how he will keep in contact with his local friends. He has no family other than a brother who lives an hour away from his semi-detached house in the town. You discuss different options, including home care and care home.

Activity 3.3   Leadership and management

1. Who should you and your Practice Supervisor involve when planning for Austin's discharge?
2. Name at least three of Austin's holistic care needs that must be considered when planning his discharge.

An outline answer is given at the end of the chapter.

Holistic care delivery

Holistic care goes beyond the biopsychosocial model of care to provide even more comprehensive support. It enables nurses to account for their patients' broader needs, including areas such as spirituality and cultural considerations (Jasemi et al., 2017).

An example of when sensitivity to a person's cultural and spiritual needs is important occurs in care after death. Lisa shares an example from her placement in the following Student Voices box.

Student voices: Lisa

I was quite emotional, but it was also a good feeling that you were getting them all tidied up for their family coming in to say their goodbyes, but it was emotional. We put all their bubble stuff and washed them and put on their perfume and washed their teeth and did their hair and put their favourite blouse on, the patient always spoke about this blouse and put their family photos close to them as well because the husband had already passed on. And they liked their teddy beside them that he had got and things like that just to make them feel more comfortable.

Lisa, 1st Year Adult Student Nurse

A quality improvement approach to reducing hospital readmissions in patients with cancer and heart failure. The challenge can be achieving holistic care within a busy setting such as a hospital ward. One way is through assessment, which helps identify patient needs, hospital rounds, flexible routines and discharge that account for the wider needs of the individual. Far more fundamental is making attempts to listen to the patient to determine their specific circumstances and needs. Try not to make assumptions or adopt a task-based approach. Instead, use each interaction as an opportunity to get to know the individual and involve them in decisions about their care.

Cultural studies are an important interdisciplinary field within the social sciences which has assisted in developing our understanding of these complex factors which intersect with wider social, political and economic aspects. From a nursing perspective, culture and spirituality can influence the determinants of health and, thus, health outcomes. It is also very important with respect to care delivery, and this is most evident in examples where a person might have different perspectives on treatments such as blood transfusions, blood transfusions and care after death. Maintaining an awareness of the various needs of people from different groups and communities can help you to ensure that the wishes of a person and their family are respected.

Activity 3.4 Reflection

A certain degree of routine is necessary within healthcare settings to help things run smoothly. However, it is essential that this is delivered in a flexible manner to support patient-centred care.

On your next placement, observe the ward's routines and see if there are any areas that could be adapted to better support patient-centred care.

How might you take forward any ideas or improvements that you identify?

An outline answer is given at the end of the chapter.

Nurses link a person's biological, social and psychological needs to provide a more comprehensive level of support for their health and wellbeing. Depending upon the setting in which the care is being delivered, this typically starts during the patient assessment when they begin their care journey. The UK consists of an increasingly older population, and with that comes frailty. Within this context, proactive and holistic care delivered close or at home is important (Lyndon et al., 2019). A holistic approach by medical and healthcare practitioners working in primary care settings is required to ensure the appropriate management and treatment of the various dimensions of frailty. Approaches such as the comprehensive geriatric assessment (CGA) can support the development of individualised care plans and support long-term follow-up in partnership with the patient and carers (British Geriatrics Society, 2019).

Case study: Bernadette and Abigail

We are now going to revisit Bernadette and Abigail from the previous chapters. Bernadette is a practising Christian who attends her local church each week and sings in its choir. Abigail does not consider herself religious, although she believes in a higher spirit and will sometimes pray. She was recently diagnosed with social anxiety after experiencing difficulties in groups that had gradually worsened. It was starting to affect her sleep and study, particularly in advance of classes and when starting a new placement area. Travelling on public transport was also causing challenges. Abigail has spoken to her personal tutor at university who directed her to Student Support services, and she will start a short counselling course soon. She also spoke with her GP online, and they discussed starting medication, although Abigail has chosen to wait and see how she gets on with the counselling. They both have busy lives caring for their young children, working and studying. Exercise and healthy eating can be a challenge due to the competing pressures on their time, although Bernadette manages to attend the gym a few times a week. Both regularly worry about their finances and have been forced on occasion to use credit cards for essential purchases. The combination of the factors above limits their opportunities to meet up with friends and family as regularly as they would like.

Activity 3.5   Critical thinking

It is not just those receiving care where consideration of holistic needs is important. It is also necessary to think about the holistic needs of those providing care. From a holistic perspective, what approaches may support Abigail and Bernadette in managing the various factors in their lives?

Think of at least one area to consider for either Abigail or Bernadette in relation to the following:

- social health;
- spiritual health;
- physical health;
- emotional health;
- psychological health.

An outline answer is given at the end of the chapter.

Cultural and spiritual considerations

Spiritual care refers to that which accounts for the individual's personal beliefs and how these give meaning and purpose to their life. This may include religious and non-religious belief systems. You should seek to understand and be respectful of your patients' beliefs. Open discussion of faith may be appropriate at these times and do not be put off if you experience some discomfort, as this is common for student nurses (Boswell et al., 2013). It may be necessary to facilitate prayer and contemplation for a patient. Many hospitals will have a multi-faith chapel or prayer room which is a quiet location where people can find space to meet their spiritual needs, like the one depicted in Figure 3.2. When on placement in a hospital setting, check if one is available and where patients can find it. It is also worth being aware that many hospitals will have a multi-faith chaplaincy service. The service can support people with their spiritual needs and help with anxieties or questions that arise while in the hospital. While this may include a person's religious requirements, the service is usually open to all, including those who are not religious.

A person's spiritual needs are often linked to their cultural needs, including their worldview, practices, norms, values and beliefs. For a description of a person's worldview, see Chapter 1. Culture refers to the shared activities and values of a group of people who live or work together. It is a community's *way of life* inclusive of shared values, behaviours and beliefs (Göl and Erkin, 2019). As a student nurse, it is important to be sensitive to other people's culture while also recognising your own values, beliefs and ideas (Matsuoka, 2021). Holistic care requires understanding patients' cultural and spiritual needs. We treat patients from diverse backgrounds, affecting their views of health, illness, treatment and care.

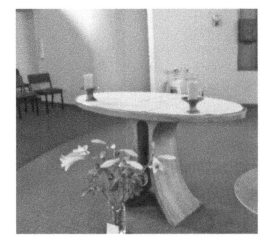

Figure 3.2 A representation of a multi-faith room

Source: iStock.com/GreenAppleNZ

Cultural sensitivity requires us to confront personal bias. Personal bias, based on one's experiences and perspectives, can creep into professional life. These biases can affect our healthcare understanding, actions and decisions. Healthcare professionals, like everyone else, have a cultural perspective. Our upbringing, experiences, values, beliefs and assumptions shape this lens, which we rarely question. Biases that prevent impartial, equitable care can be very harmful. A healthcare provider may make assumptions about a patient's beliefs or behaviour based on their own cultural norms, leading to lower-quality care (FitzGerald and Hurst, 2017). To help you overcome your assumptions, engaging in self-reflection to identify and overcome biases is useful. This requires awareness of our cultural identities, beliefs and stereotypes about other cultures. Recognising these biases helps us reduce their impact on care. It is likely that you will be encouraged to self-reflect during your nurse education, and it will also be an important feature of your future career as a registered nurse.

Empathetic care

As discussed in the previous chapter, empathy is one of the core conditions of Carl Rogers' form of humanistic psychology. One of the roots for the word 'empathy' is the German word *einfühlung*, meaning 'feeling into'. It refers to the ability to recognise the experience of another person. Empathy is key to your role as a student nurse, as it enables you to attempt to see a situation from the perspective of the person you are caring for. Transactional analysis, which we discussed in the section How Social Science Informs Holistic Care, can play a role in the development of nurses' communication and empathy skills (Whitley-Hunter, 2014). Although similar to sympathy, empathy is different insofar as you do not feel sorry for or pity the person. It allows you to develop greater sensitivity to a person's needs and can provide the basis for an enhanced therapeutic relationship with them. Demonstration of empathy can also promote other beneficial components of effective relationships, such as trust and connection. However, challenges such as organisational barriers, personal drawbacks and compassion fatigue can impede the delivery of empathetic care (Stavropoulou et al., 2020). This might be something you see for yourself while on placement.

By demonstrating empathy, nurses can improve their understanding of patient experiences and recognise any difficulties they are living through. Empathy can also work the other way, with the NMC (2022a) highlighting the public's admiration and empathy towards nurses, midwives and nursing associates, for example. Additionally, there are specific areas of nursing practice where empathy plays a more specific role. An approach in psychology focuses on *positive empathy*, which attempts to get closer to the unstated message of what the service user wants (Conoley et al., 2015, page 575). Within palliative care communications, empathy is essential, and placements in this area may provide opportunities to develop your empathetic capacity (Adriaansen et al., 2008). In the following Concept Summary, healthcare staff provide their thoughts on how to promote empathy.

Concept summary: Communication and empathy

Here are some tips that healthcare support workers submitted to the RCN (2019) to promote communication and empathy:

- *There's never too little time to care – hold a hand or lend an ear. It's the little things that count and it's what the patient remembers most.*
- *When working alongside an older person, I always imagine that they are me in the future. This teaches me to be respectful and have compassion for their vulnerability, but it also allows me to enjoy the wisdom and guidance they bestow upon me on a daily basis.*
- *Ask yourself 'how would I feel if it was me?'*

Read more here: www.rcn.org.uk/centenary/projects/100-top-tips/communication-and-empathy

As you can see, empathy is important for nurses to understand their patients' experiences and feelings. It can be supported through awareness of your own emotions and responses. This is where self-awareness and emotional intelligence are useful concepts to understand, both of which are part of the *Future nurse: standards of proficiency for registered nursing* (NMC, 2018b). Self-awareness is the conscious awareness of one's emotions, motivations, desires and personality. Self-awareness in nursing refers to understanding your emotional reactions to certain situations or patient interactions and knowing your strengths, weaknesses, biases and triggers. It is an aspect of emotional intelligence, which may be described as the ability to recognise, comprehend and manage our own emotions as well as the emotions of others (Christianson, 2020). Nurses with high emotional intelligence can navigate difficult conversations, manage stress, provide emotional support to patients and work effectively as team members. Self-awareness and emotional intelligence can help nurses be more empathic. We can be more present and aware of our patients' emotional states if we are aware of and manage our emotions. This enables us to understand their feelings and perspectives better and respond to them in a compassionate and empathetic manner.

Another way to better understand the experience of others is through reading qualitative research. Social science research includes techniques that can provide insights into patients' experiences. There are many different methods with those that explore patients' lived experiences, which you can read about in nursing and related journals. This type of research is designed to go beyond the descriptive answers someone might give when reflecting upon a situation to get closer to what it was actually like for them in the moment. The next section sets out this approach in more detail.

Lived experience

Lived experience refers to the pre-reflective experiences of an individual. It focuses on how experiences are lived rather than the descriptions of an experience. After a particular life event or situation, we often describe it in reflective terms as we process what has happened, try to make sense of it and make it fit with the wider narrative of our lives. This moves us away from the experience itself towards descriptions which are dependent upon the context we are in and who we are talking with. For example, a patient may describe their experience of a health condition differently to a healthcare professional as they might a close friend. This is a normal part of life. However, when we are truly trying to understand a person's experience, it can be worthwhile trying to get closer to what it was like for them in the moment. We can achieve this by asking questions which encourage them to talk about the experience, such as *tell me how you felt when you found out about the health condition*. The concept of lived experience has become more popular in recent years within healthcare and society more widely.

The inclusion of lived experience and the contribution of service users and experts in the design of healthcare services and education is essential. It can help us design and deliver services that are more responsive, inclusive and effective (Finn et al., 2018). When service users and their families are actively involved in services, it is easier to understand different people's needs, points of view and experiences. This can lead to new ways of giving care, a focus on the patient and better patient satisfaction and outcomes. When it comes to education, service users can give important information about the practical and emotional parts of care. These insights can help those designing the curriculum to incorporate the perspectives of patients and ultimately inform your learning as a student nurse. For example, hearing directly from a patient about what it is like to live with a chronic illness can give you valuable insight into the physical, emotional and social challenges that come with these conditions.

People who have had direct experience with a service, illness or care setting are also important in shaping and improving healthcare education (Eijkelboom et al., 2023). Their knowledge and ideas can challenge old ways of thinking and lead to new ways of caring for people. By viewing healthcare and education systems from a different angle, they can point out ways to improve them that might not otherwise be noticed. Through the inclusion of service users in the design of services and education, we make sure that their voices are heard and that their needs and preferences are met.

Chapter summary

This chapter has introduced you to the concept of holistic care. We have considered the theoretical roots of holistic care, including those originating from the social sciences. You have considered the role of empathy and the importance of developing your skills in this area. This chapter has also supported the development of understanding associated with lived experience and holistic care planning. We hope it has demonstrated to you how holistic care is an important approach within nursing practice and provided opportunities to develop your knowledge and understanding in this area. As you read the next chapter on inequalities, it is worth remembering that holistic care nursing practice can help challenge inequalities (Cowling, 2020), so look out for the links within the discussion.

Activities: Brief outline answers

Activity 3.1   Decision-making

Carolina's holistic care needs include factors such as her social relationships inside and outside of the care home, her psychological needs, particularly with respect to anxiety and depression, her emotional needs (e.g. enjoyment of the sing-along session), maintenance and promotion of her physical health, along with any religious or cultural beliefs she may have.

One approach would be to explain details about the sing-along event beforehand to prepare her for what is involved. This could be combined with meeting the professional singer in advance so there is familiarity and perhaps they could sing a song together before joining the session. Carolina could also be shown the venue and where she will sit in advance of the session beginning.

Activity 3.2   Reflection

Here are examples of things you may have considered for each area:

- Social: Nurses should be aware of my close family and friends who support and accompany me during my hospital stay.
- Physical: For personalised care, nurses must understand my physical abilities, pain levels and comfort needs.
- Emotional: Recognising my emotional reactions to hospitalisation will aid in the delivery of sensitive and compassionate care.
- Psychological: It's critical that my mental health is monitored and that any psychological issues I have are addressed.

- Spiritual: During my stay, respect and understanding for my spiritual or religious practices can provide much-needed comfort.
- Cultural: Being aware of my cultural background and practices can aid in providing respectful and culturally sensitive care.
- Environmental: The comfort and friendliness of my hospital environment can have a significant impact on my recovery and wellbeing.

Activity 3.3   Leadership and management

You should include Austin when planning his discharge. It will be important to check if Austin would like his brother or friends to participate in the discussions. It will also be necessary to involve a range of professionals, likely to include the dietician, physiotherapist, an occupational therapist (if discharged home, they can assess his home and recommend equipment to support him), a social worker to discuss care planning options and medical staff. It may also be necessary to consult other specialisms, such as pharmacists. Don't worry if you didn't get all these, but it should highlight the complexity of planning this type of discharge.

Alongside his physical care needs, such as diet and mobilisation, it will also be necessary to consider other factors including his psychological wellbeing and social circumstances.

Activity 3.4   Reflection

You could convert your thoughts and ideas into real recommendations. Focus on how these adjustments could improve patient care and possibly increase efficiency or staff wellbeing. Begin by communicating with your Practice Supervisor or Practice Assessor about your findings and comments. They have the experience to guide you and may be able to assist you in understanding the viability and potential consequences of your ideas. If appropriate, you might wish to speak with your peers as they may give similar insights, support or suggestions. Additionally, your lecturers may assist you in making professional suggestions, evaluating your observations and developing your ideas.

Activity 3.5   Critical thinking

Here are some of the holistic needs you may have considered for Bernadette:

- Social health: Competing pressures limit opportunities, although she is a church choir member.
- Spiritual health: Attends church.
- Physical health: Attends the gym a few times a week. Diet may need consideration.
- Emotional health: Bernadette appears to have minimal issues related to emotional health – although the demands on her may impact this aspect of her life.
- Psychological health: There are minimal psychological issues apparent in the information available.

Here are some of the holistic needs you may have considered for Abigail:

- Social health: Competing pressures limit opportunities for social connections.
- Spiritual health: Has non-religious beliefs.
- Physical health: Does not exercise frequently. Diet may need consideration.
- Emotional health: Abigail is likely to be experiencing emotional issues relating to her recent diagnosis. The counselling may assist with this area of her life.
- Psychological health: Recent social anxiety diagnosis may require further interventions from the GP, depending upon progress.

Further reading

Helming, MAB et al. (2020) *Dossey and Keegan's holistic nursing: a handbook for practice*. Burlington, MA: Jones and Bartlett Learning.

This text explains how holistic nursing encompasses all nursing specialities and levels, with an emphasis on theory, research and evidence-based practice.

McCormack, BT and McCance T (2016) *Person-centred practice in nursing and health care: theory and practice*. 2nd ed. Wiley-Blackwell.

This book covers the importance of person-centred care from practice, strategic and policy perspectives. It explores how this topic underpins all nursing and healthcare, including mental health services, acute care, nursing homes, community work and care for children and people with disabilities.

SCIE (2012) Common safeguarding issues – Institutionalised Care in Commissioning care homes: common safeguarding challenges. SCIE – Social Care Institute for Excellence.

This specific section of Guide 46, Commissioning care homes: common safeguarding challenges provides further information regarding institutionalised care and how to prevent it. Available at: www.scie.org.uk/publications/guides/guide46/commonissues/institutionalisedcare.asp (Accessed: 27 June 2023)

Useful websites

www.nursingtimes.net/clinical-archive/holistic-care/

The *Nursing Times* has a zone dedicated to holistic care. You can keep up to date with developments and learn more about the topic.

www.britishjournalofnursing.com/content/comment/why-its-time-to-unite-science-based-and-alternative-care-in-holistic-nursing/

This page on the *British Journal of Nursing* provides an interesting perspective on holistic care written by Sally Star, Holistic Health Practitioner.

Chapter 4　Inequalities and discrimination

Chapter aims

After reading this chapter, you will be able to:

- provide an explanation of how inequalities and discrimination apply to healthcare;
- set out the relationship between the social sciences and the topics of the chapter;
- identify and discuss examples of how to challenge diversity and inequalities;
- describe a nurse's responsibility to be inclusive and challenge discrimination as set out in the NMC (2018c) *Code of professional standards*.

Introduction

This chapter explains nurses' important role in addressing inequalities and discrimination. It provides practical examples of how nurses can recognise and challenge inequalities and discrimination wherever they encounter them. It will analyse the real-life experiences of student nurses in the practice setting to show how understanding the social sciences can ensure nurses are more attuned to both direct and indirect forms of discrimination. This will involve introducing case studies to readers to set out examples of discriminatory practices, including suggestions on responding appropriately.

Why learn about inequalities and discrimination

Student nurses care for people from all areas of society. You learn about people from across society, offering a window into how different people live. Providing care for people from diverse backgrounds during times of need has long been one of the most rewarding aspects of being a nurse. You will encounter those who have benefitted from the systems and privileges that society provides. You will also come across those disadvantaged by the societal systems and largely miss out on these benefits. While on community placement, student nurses may observe stark differences between communities in different areas while you are on placement. This will include social and economic inequalities, such as employment and income, opportunities in education and participation in society, crime levels, infrastructure, transport and housing. Health is a key area of inequality that is particularly important for you to be aware of as a student nurse.

Student voices: Carol

Carol was exposed to problems that people experience within deprived areas and how these link to unemployment, substance misuse, health inequalities and insecure family circumstances. She described a discussion with her Practice Supervisor regarding the issues they were encountering:

We talked about employment, we talked about lack of lifestyle opportunities, there are very little resources that are put into an area that could really use them, we talked about lack of education opportunities.

Carol, 2nd Year Adult Student Nurse

Economic inequalities are often aligned with inequalities in health and wellbeing (Matthews, 2015b). The UK has struggled to address health inequalities and persistent disparities have remained (Scheffer et al., 2019). The additional costs of socio-economic inequality are estimated at £4.8 billion a year in greater hospitalisations alone (NHS, 2019a). Societies with high levels of wealth and resource inequality have higher levels of poor mental and physical health across the population (UK Government, 2019). You will explore examples of these as you progress through the chapter, but let's first consider why it is important to learn about inequalities and discrimination. The NMC (2018c) standards emphasise that nurses have an essential role in reducing health equality, requiring them to work in partnership with people to develop responsive and tailored care in response to the preferences and unique circumstances of the individual. All nurses should act as an advocate for the vulnerable and treat people fairly and without discrimination (NMC, 2018c).

Activity 4.1   Reflection

Before we get into more detail in this chapter, take some time to reflect upon your next placement.

Start by asking yourself the likelihood that you will encounter people from communities and groups that experience health inequalities.

Now think of two ways to help you become more aware of the inequalities the people you encounter may be experiencing and the nurse's role in addressing them.

An outline answer is given at the end of the chapter.

What are inequalities?

Inequalities are the unequal, often unfair, distribution and delivery of resources and services among different social groups. These arise from the social and economic conditions in which people are born, live and work. McCartney et al. (2019, page 28) provide a recent definition: *Health inequalities are the systematic, avoidable and unfair differences in health outcomes that can be observed between populations, between social groups within the same population or as a gradient across a population ranked by social position.* An example of the impact of these inequalities is that people living in the least deprived areas spend a sixth of their lives in poor health, yet this jumps to nearly a third for those in the most deprived areas (UK Government, 2018a). Part of the reason for this is the higher rates of heart disease, lung cancer and chronic lower respiratory diseases within these communities.

Activity 4.2   Critical thinking

Health inequalities can involve differences across areas, such as access to care and quality of care. Think of an example of how inequalities may be a factor for each of the following:

*   health status;
*   access to care;
*   quality and experience of care;
*   behavioural risks to health;
*   wider determinants of health.

(King's Fund, 2022c)

The following website has a wealth of evidence that can help you to answer this question: www.kingsfund.org.uk/publications/what-are-health-inequalities

An outline answer is given at the end of the chapter.

These factors impact on people's lives and can significantly shorten them. During 2018–20, males in England's least deprived 10 per cent of areas could expect to live almost a decade longer than those living in the 10 per cent most deprived areas (King's Fund, 2022a). For females, the difference was eight years. National Records of Scotland (2021) show the gap in life expectancy between the most and least deprived areas in Scotland was 13.5 years for males and 10.2 years for females. The gap has widened over the past five years, growing by approximately 14 months for males and 18 months for females. The underlying reasons for these differences in health are due to a range of factors. People's mental and physical health are influenced by the wider determinants of health, incorporating a diverse range of social, economic and environmental factors (UK Government, 2018b). As mentioned earlier, the variation in these factors across groups and communities contributes to social inequality.

You may sometimes see the term 'health inequities' used instead of 'health inequalities'. Although similar, the former refers to the unfair, avoidable and remedial differences in health between different groups in society (WHO, 2021). The term 'health inequities' can be useful when highlighting systematic differences in the health status of different groups (WHO, 2018). These systemic differences often occur when people are discriminated against and face barriers to services due to protected characteristics such as race, age or sexual orientation (Heaslip et al., 2022). We use the term 'inequalities' in this chapter as it is a broader and more familiar term that often encompasses aspects of inequity.

Activity 4.3 Reflection

Hidden inequities refer to disparities or unfair situations that are not immediately visible or widely recognised. These inequities can exist in a variety of societal settings, including education, healthcare, employment and housing. They are frequently the result of systemic biases and structural barriers that disproportionately affect certain groups, such as marginalised communities, but their effects may be less widely acknowledged or understood due to their 'hidden' nature.

Reflect on the population that uses your local hospital and health services. Are there any communities or groups that may experience hidden inequities? If you are not sure, is there anything you could do to find out?

An outline answer is given at the end of the chapter.

A recent example of health inequalities and inequities at play was evident during the COVID-19 pandemic. From a global perspective, the following groups experienced an increased rate of COVID-19 morbidity and mortality:

- poorer people;
- marginalised ethnic minorities, including Indigenous Peoples;
- low-paid essential workers;
- migrants;
- populations affected by emergencies, including conflicts;
- incarcerated populations;
- homeless people.

(WHO, 2021, page iv)

The inequalities that impacted these groups during the pandemic include higher rates of chronic disease, greater exposure to the virus, barriers to engagement with public health measures and reduced access to health services. These issues are linked to the increased severity of COVID-19 and mortality rates (Pujolar et al., 2022). The disparities in chronic conditions result from differences in exposure to social determinants of health, such as living conditions, nutrition and sanitation. Frontline workers and those living in overcrowded households, often associated with lower socio-economic status, have been found to be more vulnerable to the virus (Bambra et al., 2020). Unlike those who are more affluent, people from these groups are not able to work from home or practise social isolation, which increases their risk of contracting the virus.

Case study: Bernadette and Abigail

Abigail, whom you met earlier in the book, is on a community placement in the city centre. She had heard about health inequalities and social determinants of health during her studies but had not seen them first hand. As she observes the disparities between the city's affluent and deprived areas, she begins to see the impact on the health and wellbeing of the communities. While protecting anonymity, she describes some of her experiences to Bernadette, who is on placement in the hospital. Although they both care for people from the same community, Bernadette is surprised to hear about the extent of the challenges that some people face in the local area. This had not been fully apparent as she looked after people on the ward.

Activity 4.4   Reflection

- Think of two reasons why Bernadette was not fully aware of the wider circumstances of the people she is caring for.
- What could she do to find out more about their situations?

- Why might it be an advantage for a hospital-based nurse to be aware of the circumstances in their local community?

An outline answer is given at the end of the chapter.

Leaving aside wider socio-economic factors, inequities in healthcare delivery can occur at the level of the patient, the clinical encounter, the healthcare provider, the healthcare system level (Lee and Padilla, 2022). Practical examples of factors that may impact a person's ability to access healthcare include travel costs, lost time and wage or issues relating to literacy and difficulties engaging with materials that are not accessible to them (Heaslip et al., 2022). As a nursing student, it is useful to become more aware of how inequalities can impact the health of your patients. This can help you understand and meet their needs more effectively.

Social and economic factors are the primary drivers of health outcomes and can also shape individuals' health behaviours (Artiga and Hinton, 2018). How factors combine and interact with each other can compound health inequalities. They may be influenced by the population groups to which they belong, where a person is disabled *and* from a particular ethnic background, for example. Members of the LGBTQI+ community express concerns about ageing and whether care providers will understand their needs and demonstrate anti-discriminatory practice (Taylor et al., 2021). Meanwhile, groups such as asylum seekers, refugees, and Gypsy, Roma and Traveller communities may face particular barriers (King's Fund, 2022c). How different factors combine to influence a person's opportunities and outcomes is sometimes referred to as intersectionality. People who are represented across groups such as these can face cumulative disadvantages due to the effects of intersectionality when contrasted with those who are more privileged, as shown in the following case study section.

Case study: Intersectionality

Sara is an asylum seeker from Sudan who has recently entered the United Kingdom with two young children. This case study will explore how she may encounter intersectionality in a variety of ways.

Intersectionality refers to the interconnectedness of social categories such as race, class and gender, which produce overlapping and interdependent systems of discrimination or disadvantage. In the context of a Sudanese woman with children seeking asylum, she may face multiple obstacles related to her gender, race and asylum-seeker status. First, female asylum seekers are frequently confronted with gender-specific obstacles, such as gender-based violence, trauma and difficulties in accessing appropriate healthcare. In addition, they may face discrimination and prejudice due to their race or ethnicity, which can exacerbate their

(Continued)

vulnerability (Sanders, 2019). The process of seeking asylum can be particularly difficult for women due to gender-specific issues not being adequately recognised or understood by the authorities. In addition, women with children may encounter additional obstacles when attempting to gain access to suitable housing, education and support services. The intersection of gender, race and asylum-seeking status can also have an effect on the mental health of Sudanese women and their children (Refugee Council, 2023).

We can see that a female Sudanese asylum seeker with two young children may experience intersectionality due to the challenges associated with her gender, race and asylum-seeker status. These difficulties can manifest in a variety of ways, including discrimination, access to services and mental health problems. To ensure that asylum-seeking women and their children receive the necessary support and protection, it is essential for services, including those provided by healthcare and nursing, to recognise and address these intersecting challenges.

An underlying issue that affects many disadvantaged groups is deprivation, which in turn has a detrimental impact on many health outcomes. Deprivation is apparent when quality of life is adversely affected by a lack of basic resources or necessities, such as adequate food, housing, healthcare, education and employment opportunities. Deprived communities often depend more on services and charities to meet their basic needs. People may need to access a food bank in order to feed themselves and their families for example (see Figure 4.1)

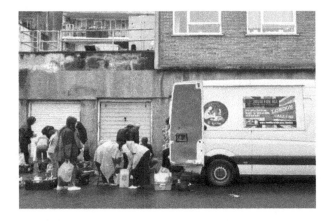

Figure 4.1 A food van delivers to vulnerable communities

iStock.com/Simon Shepheard

From the healthcare perspective, we can see how deprivation and inequalities often go hand in hand. For example, despite having high disease prevalence, deprived areas will often have fewer GPs per person and lower rates of admission for elective care (King's Fund, 2022c). Additionally, people in deprived areas are more likely to need mental health support but less likely to access it and recover following treatment (UK Government, 2019).

The disadvantages associated with deprivation and inequality can adversely affect many aspects of a person's health and wellbeing. The next section will explore the government's role in addressing these issues.

Political and government drivers

Health inequalities are a complex issue influenced by political and government drivers. Understanding these drivers will help you recognise barriers and advocate for patients and communities. A primary driver is healthcare funding. The government's allocation of budgets to the NHS directly impacts the quality and accessibility of healthcare. When resources are scarce, we see longer wait times and the possibility of service cuts. This disproportionately impacts disadvantaged communities, which may rely more heavily on public health services. The government's socio-economic strategies have a significant impact on health outcomes. These strategies include educational, employment, housing and social welfare policies. For example, austerity measures implemented in the aftermath of the 2008 financial crisis had significant health consequences, leading to increased health inequalities.

The government also shapes health inequalities through the implementation of health policy. For example, the NHS (2019a) Long Term Plan aimed to prevent and address healthcare inequalities by taking a more systematic approach to reducing unwarranted variation in care. This plan identified five key priority areas for addressing health inequalities: restoring inclusive NHS services, mitigating digital exclusion, ensuring complete and timely data sets, accelerating preventative programmes and strengthening leadership and accountability.

The role of the government in regulating the private sector can also have an indirect impact on health. Food-labelling policies, advertising of unhealthy products and pharmaceutical pricing are some examples of how government regulations can shape public health. Additionally, public health policies influence health inequalities across areas such as smoking, obesity, alcohol and drug use (The Health Foundation, 2022). If not implemented equitably, these policies aimed at improving public health can inadvertently widen health inequalities and their effects can vary across different social and economic groups. Tackling health deprivation requires working with policymakers or, from a more critical perspective, working against those holding power and influence (Scambler, 2012). As you will see in Chapter 5, this may involve lobbying against harmful policies, educating the public about health deprivation or engaging in activism. Nurses can utilise their unique position as frontline healthcare providers to give voice to those frequently unheard and help combat health inequalities.

What is discrimination?

Discrimination means treating a person unfairly as a result of who they are or because they possess certain characteristics (Equal Opportunities Commission, 2022).

The Equality Act (2010) is an important legislation that legally protects people from discrimination at work or in wider society. It includes different forms of discrimination, such as direct discrimination, when a person discriminates against another person because of a protected characteristic or treats them less favourably than others. Indirect discrimination applies when there is a discriminatory provision, criterion or practice in relation to a protected characteristic. The protected characteristics set out by the Equality Act (2010) include (a) age; (b) disability; (c) gender reassignment; (d) race; (e) religion or belief; (f) sex; (g) sexual orientation.

Concept summary: Non-discrimination

Here is an example that demonstrates when discrimination may not be considered unlawful:

A shelter for women posts an advertisement for female counsellors only. In this case, the employers could escape any potential sex discrimination complaint by arguing that all of their clients are women who have suffered domestic violence by their male partners and they would be reluctant to speak to other men about their experience.

(Equal Opportunities Commission, 2022, page 1)

Subu et al. (2021) explain that stigma refers to the social discrediting, devaluing and shaming of a person due to specific characteristics or attributes that they possess. This can lead to stigmatised people experiencing isolation, rejection, marginalisation and discrimination. The Mental Health Foundation (2021) highlights that nearly nine out of ten people with mental health problems say that stigma and discrimination negatively impact their lives. Complete Activity 4.5 to consider how these issues may affect a patient's care.

Scenario: Stigma

Imagine you are working in an orthopaedic ward. One of the nurses asks you to check on a female patient who had surgery yesterday for a badly fractured ankle. They describe the person as a *problem* patient who is being difficult with the staff. The nurse says they are asking for more medication and that he can tell the person is *exaggerating to be given stronger painkillers.*

Activity 4.5   Critical thinking

- What examples of discrimination are evident here, and what might you do in such a situation?

An outline answer is given at the end of the chapter.

An example of discrimination is the evidence that women from ethnic minority backgrounds often experience poor practice, including discrimination and cultural insensitivity when accessing maternal and neonatal services (NHS Race and Health Observatory, 2022). Women from ethnic minority backgrounds may face language barriers. This can lead to misunderstandings and miscommunications, which can result in inadequate or delayed care. In some cases, healthcare providers may fail to make adequate efforts to provide translation services, exacerbating the problem. Additionally, care providers may be unfamiliar with the cultural beliefs and practices of women of various ethnicities. This lack of cultural competence can undermine the trust and rapport required for effective healthcare delivery. To address these issues, nurses and other care providers should receive cultural competency training in order to better understand and respect their patients' diverse cultural backgrounds. Efforts should be made to recruit and retain healthcare professionals from a variety of backgrounds, as this can contribute to a more inclusive and culturally sensitive healthcare environment. Women from ethnic minority backgrounds should be encouraged to provide feedback on their healthcare experiences, raising awareness of the difficulties they face and informing the development of more inclusive healthcare.

Discrimination can be accompanied by the labelling of patients within healthcare delivery. This is where a negative label is attached to a patient by healthcare staff, influencing how they are treated. An example of this is the labelling of individuals dependent on a substance, leading to bias and the perpetuating of negative stereotypes (Valdez, 2021). Patients who are the victims of stigma and discriminatory practice can be apparent through differences in the care they receive, including patient avoidance and robotic care (Rafii et al., 2019). Wittenauer et al. (2015) explored hospital nurses' hidden attitudes concerning poverty. They found that nurses were more likely to agree with stigmatising statements than those that attributed poverty to structural factors. These examples help us to recognise that there are significant issues relating to discrimination within healthcare. The social sciences can help us explore the reasons and potential solutions for societal discrimination and inequality.

The role of the social sciences

Sociology applies a critical lens to explore society and expose inequalities. It is the discipline's central area of debate, and work carried out by the discipline applies across most areas of life, including health. Sociologists have helped to show how inequalities affect disadvantaged and marginalised groups. Theory and research methods developed by sociologists have assisted nurses in understanding of society and how inequalities impact. Many popular approaches within nursing research are termed 'social methods' and were developed by social scientists.

> ## Concept summary: City health outcomes
>
> Inequalities mean that health outcomes can vary across different parts of a country. This can also be the case across different areas of the same city. For example:
>
> In Glasgow, male life expectancy ranges from 66.2 years in Ruchill and Possilpark to 81.7 years in Cathcart and Simshill – a difference of 15.5 years. In London, when travelling east from Westminster, each tube stop represents nearly one year of life expectancy lost according to the findings of the London Health Observatory.
>
> (WHO, 2018)

Social scientists have explored how gender inequalities are manifest within the nursing profession. In many societies, nursing has traditionally been viewed as a female profession, with inherent biases and stereotypes. Female nurses frequently face challenges in leadership roles due to societal gender norms (Woolnough et al., 2019), while male nurses may face societal stereotypes that question their masculinity or competence (Taylor et al., 2022). These gender disparities can have an impact on nurses' professional development, workplace experience and mental health. We can better understand and address gender inequalities by using sociology's critical lens. Sociologists, for example, might investigate the structural barriers that prevent female nurses from advancing to leadership positions or the societal attitudes that discourage men from entering or remaining in the nursing profession. They may also look into how gender interacts with other factors like race or socio-economic status to create additional layers of inequality in nursing (Snee and Goswami, 2021).

Sociological research can also help nurses understand how gender inequalities affect health outcomes in patient care. For example, research may show that women in certain communities are less likely than men to seek help for health issues due to cultural norms. This knowledge can be used to help nurses provide more culturally sensitive, patient-centred and equitable care. Furthermore, sociological methods, also known as 'social methods' in nursing research, can be useful in investigating and addressing health disparities. These methods include qualitative techniques such as interviews and focus groups, which can capture different gender groups' lived experiences and perspectives. Quantitative methods, such as surveys and statistical analysis, can also be used to identify patterns and trends in gender inequalities. We'll look at research methods in more detail in Chapter 5.

Finally, sociology is critical in identifying and addressing gender disparities in healthcare. Nurses can gain a deeper understanding of these inequalities by applying sociological theories and methods, which can then inform their practice and contribute to more equitable health outcomes. As future nurses, you must carry on this important work by advocating for gender equality in both your professional roles and the care you provide to patients. To promote effective preventative and public health measures, those delivering services must recognise the role of social determinants

(Matthews, 2015a). This means attempting to understand the social landscape that applies to the region where you are located. Understanding the social context within which you are providing care will help you recognise the needs of groups and relevant social issues that may influence health.

Challenging inequalities – the nurse's role

As the future nursing workforce, student nurses have a vital role in addressing and reducing health inequalities. There are indications that student nurses have an awareness of health inequalities. For example, Scheffer et al. (2019) found that nursing students agree with statements promoting social justice. Social justice refers to the seeking of a society or institution founded on the principles of equality and solidarity, understands and values human rights and recognises the dignity of all people. Scheffer et al.'s (2019, page 62) study also found that student nurses disagreed with stigmatising statements towards those in poverty, such as *Welfare makes people lazy*, as well as those that emphasise personal deficiencies, such as *Poor people are dishonest*. The study shows that participants recognise the need to avoid stigmatising the people and communities they encounter when providing care.

All healthcare professionals should recognise that while lifestyle and behaviour changes can have an impact on individual health, the larger social, economic and political contexts also have a significant impact. According to Matthews (2015a), it is vital that these external influences be recognised to avoid unfairly assigning blame to those experiencing poor health due to their circumstances. Matthews (2015b) emphasises the significant impact of housing conditions and a lack of healthy, affordable food options on health outcomes, particularly in deprived areas. These conditions can contribute to health disparities, leading to many issues for those living with them. As a nursing student, you can begin to develop an understanding of how health inequalities manifest within your local area. One way to do this is to explore the socio-economic factors that impact the locality. You can do so by looking at how these are mapped across your area using measures of deprivation (see Activity 4.6).

Activity 4.6   Evidence-based practice and research

Thinking about your local area, search online for the following:

- if you are studying in Scotland: SIMD (Scottish Index of Multiple Deprivation) (https://simd.scot/);
- if you are studying in England: Indices of Deprivation 2015 and 2019 (http://dclgapps.communities.gov.uk/imd/iod_index.html);

(Continued)

- if you are studying in Wales: Welsh Index of Multiple Deprivation (full Index update with ranks) (www.gov.wales/welsh-index-multiple-deprivation-full-index-update-ranks-2019);
- if you are studying in Northern Ireland: InstantAtlas™ Report (nisra.gov.uk).

What information is available on the website for your local area? Did you learn anything – perhaps try contrasting the findings with another area you are familiar with.

An outline answer is given at the end of the chapter.

Nobody's listening

One area of concern within healthcare provision and education relates to thalassaemia and sickle cell disease. The 'No One's Listening' report is based on the findings of an investigation into preventable fatalities and healthcare failures for sickle cell patients. The All-Party Parliamentary Group (2021) released a report on sickle cell and thalassaemia in collaboration with the Sickle Cell Society. The Sickle Cell Society is a national organisation that supports and represents people affected by sickle cell disorder. The investigation reveals evidence of inferior care, inadequate training for healthcare personnel and racist attitudes. The report makes various recommendations, including the necessity for a national sickle cell and thalassaemia strategy, the formation of a national sickle cell and thalassaemia registry, and required sickle cell and thalassaemia care training for all healthcare professionals.

The report also recommends the formation of a national sickle cell and thalassaemia task force, creating a sickle cell and thalassaemia care pathway, and reviewing the current commissioning arrangements for sickle cell and thalassaemia services.

Research summary: Learning more about sickle cell disease

The Sickle Cell Society, founded in 1979, is a well-known organisation based in London and dedicated to helping sickle cell patients and their families. The organisation offers a wide range of services, including education, advocacy and support, to help people with this severe genetic disorder improve their quality of life. The Sickle Cell Society, as a major voice in the UK for sickle cell awareness, works with a variety of stakeholders, including healthcare professionals, researchers and policymakers, to promote greater understanding and enhance patient care. The organisation also raises public awareness of the condition through community outreach activities, refuting myths and encouraging early detection and management. The Sickle Cell Society plays an important role in the continuous search for better treatments and, ultimately, a cure for this life-altering disorder by creating a supportive atmosphere and investing in research. The National Heart, Lung and Blood Institute (NHLBI) website has further information about sickle cell disease. The website contains information on sickle cell disease's causes, symptoms, diagnosis, therapy and management. On the website, you may also discover information on clinical trials and research studies relating to sickle cell disease.

Raising concerns

If you encounter discrimination while on placement, it is essential that you do not wait until after the placement to raise your concerns. Your university will have a process for you to follow to raise these at the time – you can often find this in your placement paperwork or handbook. Contact your university tutor if you need further guidance. If you leave it until the placement evaluation when you have already left the placement it is often difficult for the matter to be followed up and may not benefit people being impacted by the issues.

Activity 4.7   Reflection

Follow the link below to watch a three-minute animation from the NMC which covers being inclusive and challenging discrimination. While watching, identify where nurses can get support when challenging discrimination:

www.nmc.org.uk/standards/code/code-in-action/inclusivity/

An outline answer is given at the end of the chapter.

Systemic health inequalities and discrimination

The NHS comes into contact with over a million people every 24 hours (NHS, 2019a). The provision of this level of health service, free to the vast majority of people at the point of service, can broadly be viewed as a social good. It is certainly a system that many people value in the UK and prefer over other systems where people pay directly or through private insurance. Unlike the NHS, people reliant upon these systems who lack the economic means can be denied the care they would receive in the UK. Despite the benefits of the NHS for society, it nonetheless is prone to systemic inequalities and discrimination. We'll now explore areas where you may encounter these issues as a nursing student.

Encountering discrimination on placement

It is important that you demonstrate an inclusive and non-discriminatory approach while providing care. This involves recognising and respecting individual rights and preferences. These include those associated with gender identity, ethnicities, sexual orientation, religion and belief, age, disabilities, and socio-economic background, many of which are protected characteristics under equality legislation. In a healthcare setting, discrimination can have damaging effects on patient care. Patients who encounter discrimination are more likely to experience negative feelings, including anxiety, depression, disappointment and shock, with discriminatory nursing likely to be harmful to their health and wellbeing (Rafii et al., 2019).

Activity 4.8   Evidence-based practice and research

In the section What Is Discrimination? the two different types of discrimination were introduced: direct and indirect discrimination. Look at the following scenarios from an acute healthcare setting.

- A patient is treated unfairly – is this direct or indirect discrimination?
- A patient is avoided – is this direct or indirect discrimination?

An outline answer is given at the end of the chapter.

The NMC (2018c) highlights that nurses should challenge any discriminatory attitudes and behaviours they encounter. So how can you put this into action? The first thing to highlight is that you have the right to challenge discrimination then and there (NMC 2020b). Discussing your concerns with your Practice Supervisor or Practice Assessor should provide opportunities for you to receive support with the situation. It might also be appropriate to speak with the nurse in charge of the area in which you are on placement. Student experiences of discrimination from healthcare professionals and educators can undermine confidence and reduce their motivation (Jazi et al., 2022). If a satisfactory resolution is not forthcoming, the next step is to contact the university who will have a process for managing issues of this nature.

Cox et al. (2021) highlight the issue of hair discrimination within nursing. The authors point out that there is a lack of awareness about the deep cultural and historical significance of Black people's hair. They describe examples of racist behaviours, such as being told to tame the hair or wash freshly washed hair prior to the next day. A compelling case is advanced by Cox et al. (2021) for the urgent need to challenge the policies and practices associated with hair discrimination within nursing.

Brathwaite et al. (2022) discuss the historical roots of nursing, its Victorian ideals of the late eighteenth century, and the forms of discrimination that these incorporated.

This included anti-Black discrimination, alongside others, such as sexism and classism. Perceived discrimination against staff by peers can lead those affected to dislike their job and profession, accompanied by an increased desire to leave (ZareKhafri et al., 2022). Discriminatory attitudes may also arise from interactions with patients. It is worth remembering patients may be stressed or confused, and their illness may impact their ability to communicate. However, it is still okay to let them know how you feel and that it is unacceptable. Be clear with the person and explain why you want them to change their behaviour, ensuring that you keep a record of the interactions (NMC, 2020b).

Chapter summary

In this chapter, you have learned about inequalities in society and how these can impact the health of individuals and their communities. You have been introduced to an example where health services have failed to deliver care equitably. The social sciences have an important role in highlighting the inequalities in society and finding ways to address them. This includes understanding the different forms of discrimination as well as a student nurse's role in challenging these. The next chapter will build upon this to consider how nurse activism can bring about positive change for nurses and the communities with whom they provide care.

Activities: Brief outline answers

Activity 4.1   Reflection

During your next placement in a community or hospital setting, you will almost certainly come into contact with people from communities and groups who face health inequalities. Here are two examples of how you can become more aware of the inequalities that the people you encounter may be experiencing. Firstly, you could undertake some online research to learn about the common inequalities that various populations face within the local area, such as those related to race, ethnicity, socio-economic status, gender or age. Secondly, you could develop your cultural competency skills by actively listening to your patients, empathising with their experiences and respecting their beliefs and values.

Activity 4.2   Critical thinking

- Health status: Disparities in health outcomes can result from health inequalities, with marginalised populations frequently experiencing higher morbidity and mortality rates.
- Access to care: Inequalities in healthcare access can be caused by factors such as geographic location, income or insurance status, affecting vulnerable groups disproportionately.
- Quality and experience of care: Health inequalities can contribute to differences in the quality of care received and patient experiences, with certain populations facing discrimination or inadequate treatment.
- Behaviour risks to health: Social and economic disparities may expose people to higher levels of behavioural risks, such as tobacco use, poor nutrition or a lack of physical activity.
- Wider determinants of health: Health inequalities can be exacerbated by factors such as education, employment, income and living conditions, among others.

Activity 4.3   Reflection

Here are examples of communities or groups that may be affected by hidden inequities. Racial and ethnic minorities may receive lower-quality healthcare and face more barriers to access.

Language barriers can lead to misunderstandings, misdiagnoses and overall lower quality of care for immigrants or non-English speakers. The LGBTQI+ Community may face discrimination, judgement or misunderstanding, leading to inadequate care. People with disabilities can experience barriers to access, and other forms of discrimination can contribute to healthcare disparities for this population.

If you're unsure about potential hidden inequities in your community, you can speak with your Practice Supervisor (in placement) or lecturers to learn more. Find out what local services are doing to reduce inequities and try looking at local demographic data on health outcomes or access to healthcare services in your area.

Activity 4.4   Reflection

Bernadette may lack awareness as she has had fewer opportunities to observe the wider social context in which her patients live. Due to the setting, she may not have been able to engage in deeper conversations with her patients, making it more difficult for her to gain insight into their personal lives, backgrounds and the challenges they face in their communities. To find out more about their circumstances, Bernadette could ask those who have worked directly with the community to develop a more in-depth understanding of patients' social situations and can provide valuable insights. This could include social workers, occupational therapists and community nurses involved with the patients she cares for. A hospital-based nurse will benefit from an understanding of the circumstances in their local community as it will enable them to provide more comprehensive and tailored care, taking into account patients' social circumstances and the unique challenges they may face. They will be better placed to identify and address potential barriers to care.

Activity 4.5   Critical thinking

Several instances of discrimination are evident in this situation. One example is the issue of labelling. Instead of focusing on understanding the underlying reasons for the patient's requests, the nurse labels the patient as a *problem* patient, which implies a negative connotation and judgement about the patient's behaviour. Another example is that the nurse's comment about the patient wanting stronger pain relievers may suggest a stereotype that patients with certain conditions or backgrounds are more likely to engage in drug-seeking behaviour. In these circumstances, it is important to approach the patient with an open mind and actively listening to their concerns allows you to listen empathetically. Recognise their pain and discomfort and ask questions to learn more about their experience and needs. If you believe that a patient is being treated unfairly or that there is discrimination, discuss it with your Practice Supervisor and seek guidance from your university as appropriate.

Activity 4.6   Evidence-based practice and research

You may have discovered that particular locations are more disadvantaged in some domains than others. Comparing different areas might help you better understand how deprivation affects various aspects of living in different places. Here is a summary of the information available via each of the platforms:

- Scottish Index of Multiple Deprivation (SIMD): This tool analyses deprivation in different Scottish regions. It shows local deprivation related to income, employment, health, education, skills and training, housing, geographic access and crime.
- Deprivation Indices: This index, like SIMD, measures deprivation in tiny areas across England. It examines income, employment, education, health, disability, crime, housing and service barriers, and living environment deprivation.
- Welsh Index of Multiple Deprivation: Measures relative deprivation in local Welsh districts. Income, employment, health, education, access to services, community safety, physical environment and housing are covered.
- InstantAtlasTM (nisra.gov.uk): This interactive website includes Northern Ireland statistics and indicators across domains.

Activity 4.7 Reflection

The video highlights that nurses have the right to ask their managers and leaders for help and support with challenging discrimination. Support can also be found via organisations such as trade unions and relevant charities.

Activity 4.8 Evidence-based practice and research

The first is an example of direct discrimination if they are being treated unfairly because of their race, ethnicity, gender, age, disability, sexual orientation or other protected characteristics.

In terms of avoiding a patient, this is also an example of direct discrimination if they are being deliberately avoided due to protected characteristics.

It is important to note that unconscious discrimination may play a role in both situations, as it may be based on unconscious biases or stereotypes towards certain groups.

Further reading

Marmot, M (2015) *The health gap: the challenge of an unequal world*. London: Bloomsbury.

The social determinants of health and the impact of health inequalities on individuals and communities in the United Kingdom and around the world are discussed in this book.

Olusoga, D (2017) *Black and British: A forgotten history*. London: Picador Books.

Although not specifically focused on healthcare, this book provides valuable insights into the experiences of Black people in Britain and can help you to understand the historical context of racial inequalities and discrimination in the UK.

Useful websites

NHS Health Scotland: **www.healthscotland.scot**/

NHS Health Scotland offers resources and publications on health inequalities and the social determinants of health in Scotland.

King's Fund: **www.kingsfund.org.uk**/

It is a non-profit organisation that works to improve health and care in England. Use its website to find resources, research and publications on a variety of topics, including health disparities and healthcare discrimination.

The Health Foundation: **www.health.org.uk**/

This is an independent charity dedicated to improving healthcare quality in the UK. They provide resources and research on health inequalities and other related issues.

The Race Equality Foundation: **https://raceequalityfoundation.org.uk**/

The Race Equality Foundation is a non-profit organisation that promotes racial equality in a variety of fields, including healthcare. They provide information and publications about healthcare disparities and discrimination.

The Equality Trust: **www.equalitytrust.org.uk**/

The Equality Trust is an organisation that works to reduce income inequality and its consequences. They offer research, resources and information on health inequalities and their connection to income inequality.

Chapter 5 Activism and politics

Chapter aims

After reading this chapter, you will be able to:

- provide an explanation of activism;
- explain the benefits of nurses engaging in activism;
- set out the nurse's role with respect to activism;
- consider professional and ethical considerations;
- identify and discuss examples of how to engage in activism.

Introduction

This chapter will provide the knowledge to help you understand and engage in activism. It starts by reviewing what the term 'activism' means and exploring its historical context with respect to nursing. Understanding the political context will enable you to better recognise opportunities for influence and collaboration, improving your capacity to bring about positive changes for patients, communities and wider society. You will explore practical techniques and resources that can assist you in participating in nurse activism and politics, both as individuals and as part of a collective. In addition, there will be a discussion of ethical and professional considerations, including issues that nurses may encounter while participating in activism and political activities. The chapter will assist you in expanding on your current knowledge so that you are prepared to become a more proactive and influential student nurse.

What is activism?

Activism may be defined as a co-ordinated attempt by individuals or groups to effect social, political or environmental change, frequently in response to perceived injustices or inequality. It includes various activities such as peaceful protests, lobbying, grassroots organising, awareness campaigns, direct action and civil disobedience. Activists may advocate for human rights, social justice, environmental protection or political reform to influence public opinion, policy and legislation. Activism can take many forms, ranging from solitary acts to major movements, and it can involve people from many walks of life. For example, experiences of disability, loneliness or abuse were concealed, covered up and ignored before being uncovered and made public due to impassioned activism (Mulgan, 2019). It is frequently motivated by the notion that individuals have the ability and obligation to challenge and change the status quo and that collective action can have a substantial and long-term influence. Individuals and groups who engage in activism hope to bring attention to vital issues, motivate others to join their cause, and ultimately create a more just and equal society. Activism aims to challenge and change existing structures, policies or attitudes to make society fairer.

Concept summary: Roots of activism

The roots of activism may be traced back to the Romans and other ancient cultures. Roman citizens would gather in public forums and make speeches to lobby for their rights, influence decision-makers and shape government policy (Florell, 2021).

Social movements have an elusive power but one that is altogether real.

(Tarrow, 2022, page i)

Over the past couple of decades, the methods of activism have been transformed, as connectivity and social media have radically changed activists' ability to connect, organise and have an impact. However, Shaw (2013) argues that the fundamental principles for winning struggles have not changed. These principles are based upon the belief that change is possible and a willingness to carry out courageous acts in the face of opposition. You will explore some examples as you progress through later sections.

Why learn about activism?

Reading this chapter will provide insights into the different forms of activism and the benefits change can bring. You will explore examples of how activism may contribute to the continual improvement of healthcare, improving the lives of nurses and the people and communities for whom they care. Activism is one way that marginalised populations can achieve equity and social justice. Nurses can assist by advocating for their patients to challenge and address issues such as discrimination, racism and disparities in healthcare outcomes. They can also engage in activism to raise awareness about the significance of the nurse's role in society and help to advance the profession.

Activity 5.1   Reflection

Read the following passage from Jean Watson, Founder and Director of the Watson Caring Science Institute:

> *Nursing has a global covenant with humanity, to sustain human caring, healing, health, and wholeness for humanity; in instances where human caring is threatened, be it biological or otherwise.*

> (Watson, 2020, page 701)

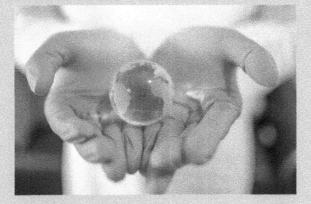

Figure 5.1   A representation of nursing's covenant

Source: iStock.com/Zephyr18

Note your initial thoughts when you have read the statement. Think about what these words mean to you as a nursing student and your role within the profession. Does it capture the nursing profession's fundamental responsibility and dedication to promoting and maintaining people's wellbeing worldwide?

An outline answer is given at the end of the chapter.

As a nursing student, you will have unique opportunities to gain intimate insights into many people's lives in a way that goes beyond that which most people in society will experience. This perspective allows you to understand the challenges and inequalities people face during their lives and recognise improvements that can help support their health and wellbeing. Nurses tend not to see their efforts as activism (Ojemeni et al., 2023) and could more fully recognise their influence across micro (individual), meso (organisational) and macro (societal) levels (Arabi, 2014). We can see that nurses advocate for their individual patients at a micro level by advocating for patients' rights, guiding them through the healthcare system or working with other providers to meet their needs. Advocating for organisational changes is meso-level activism. A nurse may advocate for safer staffing ratios or lead a team to implement evidence-based protocols in their department. At the macro level, nurse activism affects the healthcare system and society at large. This could involve lobbying for health policy reforms, public health campaigns or health inequality awareness.

It is crucial that student nurses understand the significance of developing effective leadership skills in nursing (Major, 2019). This is because it plays a vital role in improving patient outcomes and enhancing the quality of care. The NMC (2018c) *Code of professional standards* emphasises the importance of leadership and establishes clear expectations for behaviour and practice. Activism and leadership often go hand in hand as interconnected aspects that can shape patient care, nursing practice and the healthcare landscape. As highlighted in Activity 5.1, the heart of nursing is a commitment to the wellbeing of patients. Activism, then, can be seen as an extension of this commitment. It involves identifying the issues that impact patient health and wellbeing – from institutional policies to societal health disparities – and using one's voice, influence and actions to effect change. As you read through the remainder of this chapter, keep in mind that your voice as a nurse can be influential. Both in terms of those you interact with and also in the wider sense of nursing's role in society.

Nursing activism

The concept of nursing activism develops out of the ethical duties and social contract with humanity inherent to the nursing profession. Florell (2021, page 138) defines nursing activism as *requiring the expenditure of personal energy and social or political capital to address upstream and downstream determinants of health.*

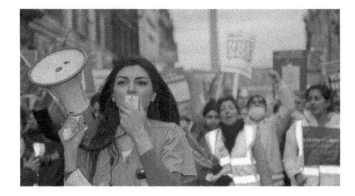

Figure 5.2   Healthcare staff protesting

Source: John Gomez / Shutterstock

This quote from Florell (2021) tells us that nursing activism is about doing something tangible to have an impact. Nurses can engage in activism in a wide range of situations, often to address inequalities and improve outcomes. All nurses have a role in promoting inclusivity and helping to dismantle systemic barriers that impact marginalised groups (Brathwaite et al., 2022). Promoting diversity enhances culturally competent care and better serves patients from a wide range of backgrounds. Nursing activism may apply locally, such as seeking to improve access to local services, to national campaigns and global issues such as climate change. Professional concerns such as patient safety, fair pay and workforce circumstances can also motivate nursing activism.

Student voices: From Zauderer et al., 2008, page 7

It is a professional responsibility to be aware of issues that affect nursing, and to take actions for change.

Nursing activism strives to promote the voices of nursing professionals to ensure their viewpoints influence policymaking, legislation and public discourse. It can take a variety of forms, ranging from individual acts of advocacy to collaborative efforts by professional organisations and unions. We'll look at examples of different forms of activism throughout this chapter. Nurses can make a difference in the areas they are passionate about by engaging with decision-makers, participating in public debates and establishing awareness campaigns. Protesting can be appropriate in some circumstances, although there can be ethical and professional considerations (there is a section on this later in the chapter). Protests are public demonstrations where people gather to show their opposition or support for a cause. They can take several forms, such as marches, sit-ins and picketing. These can enable nurses to draw attention to an issue, pressure decision-makers and influence public opinion.

Concept summary: Advocacy vs activism

Patient advocacy promotes patients' rights, needs and interests. This includes advocating for patients' access to proper medical care, defending their rights and autonomy and respecting their voices in healthcare choices. Healthcare professionals, family, friends and patient advocacy groups can advocate for patients. Patient advocacy includes helping people navigate the healthcare system or lobbying for a treatment plan. It may also involve campaigning for policy changes or enhancing vulnerable groups' access to healthcare. Patient advocacy is crucial in nursing since nurses often interact with patients first. Nurses can represent their patients and increase healthcare quality and accessibility. Patient advocacy helps nurses help patients navigate the healthcare system and get the best care. Nurses must protect patients' rights and voices in healthcare decisions.

Patient advocacy promotes patients' rights, needs and interests. This includes advocating for patients' access to care, supporting their rights and autonomy and respecting their voices in healthcare choices. Nurses, family, friends and patient groups can all advocate for patients. Patient advocacy includes helping people navigate the healthcare system or lobbying for a specific treatment or service. In similarity to nurse activism, it may also involve campaigning for policy changes or enhancing vulnerable groups' access to healthcare.

Patient advocacy is a recognised aspect of nursing care and can also be an integral component of activism. However, the latter is required to bring the necessary energy and disruption for systemic changes (Florell, 2021). While advocacy is essential for improving care for individuals and groups of patients, it often does not go far enough to bring about systemic changes. This is where nurse activism can have a greater impact.

Another way that nurses can engage in activism is through lobbying. This involves personally contacting politicians and policymakers in order to influence their decisions and pass on your views on a topic. Often it is useful to gather support for the cause through grass-roots organising in which a community of like-minded nurses come together to work together towards change and empowerment. While one nurse contacting a politician may have an impact, the lobbying is likely more effective if a group of nurses lobby together. For example, if you are a nurse concerned about Mental Health Services, you could begin by gathering evidence on the subject before rallying support from like-minded colleagues. Once organised, your group can approach local politicians with a clear message backed up by evidence, urging them to improve mental health services. Grass-roots activists often use this approach alongside other methods, such as community meetings, door-to-door discussions and public forums to try to win support for their cause. They often focus on local concerns and involve people in decision-making processes. Collective action, informed by your unique perspective as a healthcare professional, can be a powerful tool for bringing about positive change.

Nurses can also use awareness campaigns to inform the public about specific topics or causes. This is typically achieved through mainstream media, social media or public events. Social media campaigns are among the most common approaches for raising awareness. You might have encountered hashtag campaigns on social media as an example. Another approach that nurse activists may use is online or in-person petitioning. Petitioning involves gathering supporters' signatures to demonstrate public support for a given cause. These raise awareness and can be passed to government officials or organisations to pressure them to bring about positive change. This section has explored examples of how nurses may be involved in activism. These approaches can assist nurses in bringing about change in the areas that they are passionate about.

Activity 5.2   Evidence-based practice and research

Choose a topic you are interested in related to the nursing profession or health inequalities. Here are a few examples: safe staffing levels, reducing inequalities in the delivery of a local health service and reducing financial stress on nursing students. Next, choose a form of activism that you think would be most effective in addressing the issue:

- protests;
- lobbying politicians;
- grass-roots organising;
- awareness campaigns.

Finally, provide a couple of sentences on why you chose that form of activism.

An outline answer is given at the end of the chapter.

The approaches discussed in this chapter can help nurses bring about change in the areas they are passionate about. Nurses are well placed to understand people and communities in a manner that is unique to the profession. They can develop a deep understanding of the changes required to improve the lives of those they provide care for. Engaging in activism enables nurses to improve the health service and address the determinants that affect patients and their communities. In this manner, nurses can have an important role in promoting equality and social justice. They can take steps to address issues such as discrimination, racism and inequality in healthcare access and outcomes by addressing these concerns. Nurses can engage in activism to raise awareness about the value of their work in the healthcare industry and the nursing profession in general in order to advance the nursing profession. Before we move on to examples of nurse activism, it is important to emphasise that the NMC (2018c) professional code of conduct and ethical standards of the nursing profession should guide any activism you engage with.

Examples of nurse activists

Nursing activism has a long history of pushing for improvements in healthcare, social reform and the nursing profession itself. Nursing's role in fighting for change even stretches beyond the bounds of the profession to wider social issues. Nurses have been involved in fighting for *women's right to vote, laws against child labour, factory and garment worker welfare, unionisation, vaccination, housing reform, humane treatment of mentally ill people, birth control, and the control of nursing education, registration, and practice* (Fowler, 2017, page 1). Indeed, the fight for women's suffrage in 1918 included active participation from nurses (RCN, 2023). Over time many nurse activists have brought about positive change, often in difficult circumstances. We'll now consider several examples of nurse activists who have made a difference.

The first is Dame Cicely Saunders, who founded St Christopher's Hospice in 1967. It was the first hospice to link expert pain and symptom control, compassionate care, teaching and clinical research (St Christopher's, 2023). These developments led to many improvements in the field of palliative care. The second example is Dame Elizabeth Anionwu, who played a central role in several key nursing developments. Despite facing many barriers due to her mixed-race heritage, she was instrumental in establishing a groundbreaking sickle cell service that led to a national screening programme for the condition. She was also a key figure in the successful campaign to honour Black nurse Mary Seacole with a statue in St Thomas' Hospital grounds (Agnew, 2016). Both Dame Cicely Saunders and Dame Elizabeth Anionwu nurses significantly impacted their fields through passion and perseverance. While the history of nursing is steeped in social and political activism, it is worth noting that it is often downplayed in contemporary nursing (Florell, 2021). At times this is due to a blurring of the distinction between 'activism' and 'advocacy' (see Concept Summary: Advocacy vs Activism). Nurse activists can bring meaningful improvements to healthcare and society to build upon the successes of the past.

A well-known nursing activist is Linda Bailey. She believes that nurses have a unique role to play in combatting climate change. In an interview with the *Nursing Times* (Devereux, 2022), she stressed the importance of nurses in increasing awareness about the link between climate change and its negative consequences on human health. She spoke with people who had heart failure, atrial fibrillation, cellulitis and leg ulcers as a result of the severe heat and increased physiological stress on their bodies. Ms Bailey believes that nurses may use their personal observations and interactions with patients to highlight the tangible effects of the climate catastrophe on health, transforming them into potent agents of change in the fight against climate change. We can see in this example that the motivation for activism is concern regarding risks to human health and welfare. However, it is worth remembering that advocating for the environment is emotional labour, and nurses who practice environmental activism require both practical and emotional support from their colleagues (Terry and Bowman, 2020). Having support enables nurse environmental activists to continue fighting for community and global health.

Getting involved

As a student nurse, you can impact social and political circumstances that affect your patients and communities. You can advocate for change, create awareness, educate others and influence policy in a different area of health (Sweeney, 2022). Your lecturers can serve as role models in encouraging students to acquire and sustain an active knowledge of and participation in determining public policy. Learning opportunities that require nursing students to get politically involved can help them recognise the power and importance of their views (Zauderer et al., 2008). Through avenues such as social media, student nurses can connect with other activists, share knowledge and mobilise action.

Case study: Bernadette and Abigail

Bernadette, whom we have met in previous chapters, was looking forward to her placement at a nearby hospital. During Bernadette's first week, her Practice Supervisor assigned her to care for Mr Johnson, an older adult who had recently undergone surgery. Upon entering his room, Bernadette identified herself as his nurse for the day, but Mr Johnson demanded a different nurse and directed a racial slur towards Bernadette. Despite her pain, she kept her cool and notified her Practice Supervisor about the concerning events. The issue was escalated appropriately, and senior staff challenged the patient's behaviour and supported Bernadette. Bernadette's university was contacted to provide follow-up support.

Bernadette's friend Abigail notices her friend is upset and offers support. She is shocked by her friend's experiences; they seem so different from how patients interacted with her during the first week. Bernadette says she wants to do something so other students do not have to go through the same experience. Abigail suggests that she speak with the Student Union to discuss how she can become involved in activism. The Student Union has a group focused on improving the experiences of Black students. Bernadette became actively involved in the group, and they now liaise with those responsible for the nursing curriculum at the university. By raising awareness of experiences of racism, the policy for supporting students who encounter discrimination is updated. This results in a joint campaign designed to improve staff and patient awareness that racism will not be tolerated under any circumstances.

Activity 5.3   Critical thinking

- Can you think of any other sources of support that Bernadette could seek to help with her cause?
- Do you think Abigail did the right thing by suggesting that Bernadette become involved in activism? Consider if there are any pros and cons.

An outline answer is given at the end of the chapter.

Using social media, you can keep yourself politically informed, seek to improve social justice and engage in public debate (Gregory et al., 2022). When used effectively, social media can be a powerful tool for influencing political discourse, policymaking and global movements, all while inspiring people to find their voice online and offline (Gregory et al., 2022). The NMC has guidance related to social media use, and you can read more in the ethical and professional considerations section later in this chapter. Nurses can keep their profession and the health of their communities relevant by using social media to advocate for social justice and influence public debate. Engaging with social media can be time consuming and may conflict with other pressures like classes, exam preparation, essays, work and family responsibilities. For this reason, it is important to ensure that you engage with activism in a way that fits with your schedule and does not present too much stress.

Scenario: Activism

Imagine being a final-year nursing student. You've always been passionate about both healthcare and the environment. You find an article on the healthcare industry's environmental impact while researching your essay. You are surprised to learn that the sector generates substantial greenhouse gas emissions, waste and unused resources. You decide to investigate further. Your lecturers and peers share your concern and want to learn more, so you start there.

You discover that the healthcare sector can reduce its ecological footprint by cutting waste, employing renewable energy and improving supply chain management. You initiate a campus-wide healthcare sustainability campaign to make a difference. Your university supports your outreach to local healthcare practitioners to promote environmentally friendly practices. With support from colleagues, you reach out to a local expert in sustainability to talk at a seminar on the topic.

Activity 5.4   Reflection

What else could you do to promote environmental issues in nursing and healthcare?

An outline answer is given at the end of the chapter.

Depending on their specific areas of expertise and interests, registered nurses in the United Kingdom have numerous opportunities to participate in political and social activities. Student nurses can volunteer their time with local organisations such as free clinics or food banks to participate in community service activities. You can also hold health fairs or participate in public education initiatives to raise community awareness of health issues. You could get involved by joining a political party and working to change policy or lobbying for issues that are important to you. If you do not wish to join a party, you could write to your local member of parliament about a nursing-related topic that you are passionate about. Attending marches and demonstrations is another way to raise awareness and advocate for change.

Activity 5.5   Reflection

Create a mind map to visually represent the areas of society you are passionate about (e.g. mental health, environmental justice, social determinants of health).

Draw branches from each passion, listing specific changes you would like to see in these areas to improve the health and wellbeing of people and communities.

Now choose one area to research online to discover if any nurse activism is related to the topic.

An outline answer is given at the end of the chapter.

Student nurses can engage in activism by raising awareness of critical health issues through social media. You could create and share information with the goal of educating the general public on a particular subject. This could also involve participating in online forums and groups to interact with others working on similar topics. Student nurses' use of social media is a powerful tool for activism.

Ethical and professional considerations

Nurses have a trusted voice that can influence the public's awareness and perception of a topic (Devereux, 2022). Nurses can use their voice to raise awareness and foster public sympathy towards issues of concern, such as challenging inequalities or raising awareness of environmental issues. This brings both power and responsibility. The NMC (2018c) *Code of professional standards* should guide nurses' activism. When campaigning for a particular cause, you must be aware of the risks and benefits of activism and whether it is aligned with the NMC (2018c) code. You should avoid engaging in discriminatory or harassing behaviour, and respect the independence of individuals and communities. It is also worth being aware of any potential conflicts of interest and taking time to consider the impact of their activism on your colleagues and the wider profession.

Activism is rarely referred to within nursing's guidelines and standards, with Buck-McFadyen and MacDonnell (2017) arguing that this demonstrates the muted and often contested nature of activism within the profession. Nurses that engage in activism can feel isolated and overwhelmed (Terry and Bowman, 2020). Support from fellow nurses can help mitigate these feelings, but it is important to understand the benefits and risks of activism at a personal level. Regardless of how important you perceive an issue, others may see it differently and encounter political resistance to activism and even hostility (Mulgan, 2019). Being realistic about the potential challenges you may encounter and developing resilience can assist when seeking change in an important area.

The NMC (2022b) advises nurses on how to use social media. According to the guidelines, nurses should always use social media with professional boundaries and should not post anything that could bring the nursing profession into disrepute. They should also be aware of the risks to patient confidentiality when using social media and should not post any identifiable information about patients without their express consent. Furthermore, nurses should not use social media to make disparaging or offensive remarks about colleagues, patients or other people, and they should not engage in online bullying or harassment. They should also be aware of the possibility of online interactions escalating into real-life conflicts and take precautions to avoid this. Nurses are also advised to be mindful of their own mental health and wellbeing when using social media and to take precautions to protect themselves from online abuse or harassment.

Concept summary: Trade unions

A trade union is a collection of workers who have come together to negotiate better working conditions, pay and other benefits with their employer. These unions aim to improve working conditions, protect employees from exploitation and secure a fair wage for everybody. Nurses may join many unions within the UK, depending on whether they work in clinical, educational or private settings. We'll now focus on the role of two unions that are popular with nurses.

The RCN is the largest nursing professional organisation in the United Kingdom. Through its political action committee, the RCN is dedicated to advancing the nursing profession and the interests of its members. It advocates for policies that benefit nurses and their patients, such as adequate staffing levels, equitable pay and safe working conditions (RCN, 2023). Furthermore, the RCN conducts research and critical analysis on major issues affecting the nursing profession and uses the results to inform its advocacy efforts. This can include studies on the effects of government policies on the nursing workforce or the effects of social determinants of health on patient outcomes. The RCN also offers its members a variety of tools and training to help them participate in lobbying and advocacy activities. These can be a great starting point if you are interested in contributing to issues that impact nurses and those in their care.

Activity 5.6   Critical thinking

Members of nursing unions have recently been on strike for the first time in many years as they attempt to improve pay and conditions. You may have seen this reported in the news and perhaps heard about it during your studies.

(Continued)

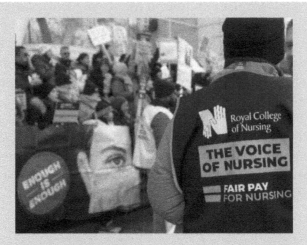

Figure 5.3   RCN members on strike

Source: John Gomez / Shutterstock

Answer the following questions:

- Do you agree or disagree with the strikes? Explain your answer.
- Evaluate the impact the campaigns to improve pay will have impacted the public perception of nurses. Provide at least one positive and one negative impact.
- What reasons may influence your decision to vote strike or not once you become a registered nurse? Explain your answer.

An outline answer is given at the end of the chapter.

UNISON is another union that also represents nurses and other healthcare professionals. UNISON's (2019) mission is to give its nursing members support and representation, including employment advice, legal representation and training, and development opportunities. In common with the RCN, UNISON also advocates for better working conditions and remuneration on behalf of its members. A recent example of this is union activity to improve nurses' pay and conditions. This resulted in the government and key healthcare unions reaching an agreement on a compensation proposal that includes a wage increase and a one-off sum. However, many nurses remain upset that the increase is significantly below inflation in the UK. As you may have discovered when completing Activity 5.6, striking is a controversial topic within nursing, with many holding different views on the topic. Some nurses feel opposed to striking because of the potential impact on patients, while others feel it is essential to ensure the voice of nurses is heard (Essex and Weldon, 2022). Leaving aside the controversy of strikes, healthcare unions play an important role in highlighting the concerns of nurses and campaigning for change.

Representation

A lack of under-represented groups in nursing and healthcare negatively affects patient care, supervision opportunities and leadership positions. Due to the evolving nature of healthcare and the focus on patient-centred care, there is a great need for nurses to be included on hospital and health boards (Disch and Kingston, 2021). This can positively influence patient care and improve organisational performance. An example where representation is important is on the board that oversees individual health organisations and services. A representative board is better equipped to understand and respond to the unique health needs of various cultural and ethnic groups. This can help ensure that health services are culturally sensitive and inclusive by having members familiar with different communities. Additionally, members of the community should have a say in decisions affecting their health and wellbeing. Boards can ensure accountability to the population they serve by including members from different backgrounds. Doing so is more likely to inspire public trust and confidence, increasing engagement and participation in health services.

Another important area of representation is within senior leadership teams. Despite the fact that women make up the majority of the healthcare workforce in the United Kingdom, they are significantly under-represented in leadership positions. Consider the NHS, where women account for 75 per cent of the workforce but continue to be poorly represented in senior positions. This disparity is not limited to the United Kingdom. While women make up 70 per cent of health workers worldwide, they hold only 26 per cent of representative positions (Pérez-Sánchez et al., 2021). Women are less common higher up the leadership hierarchy, and those of colour face even greater inequalities. Diverse leadership fosters a broader range of perspectives, which can result in more effective and innovative solutions, ultimately improving patient care.

Chapter summary

During this chapter, you have explored the concept of activism. You have learned how nurses can use activism to influence healthcare policy, improve patient care and address health disparities. This includes the historical and ongoing role that nurses have played in advocating for better patient care, better working conditions and more equitable healthcare systems. Several influential nurse activists were introduced, showing how nurses can contribute significantly to social and political change. We hope the chapter has shown how nursing students can participate in activism on a variety of levels, from local community initiatives to national efforts. It has provided you with ways to identify important issues and find ways to contribute your unique perspectives and skills. This chapter has helped you to understand the significance of political engagement and advocacy in their profession.

(Continued)

This can help you to shape a more equitable, compassionate and effective health-care system for all. Here is a final thought on the topic from a nurse activist:

It took me quite a long time to develop a voice, and now that I have it, I am not going to be silent.

(Madeleine Albright, cited in Florell 2021)

Activities: Brief outline answers

Activity 5.1   Reflection

It could be argued that the statement implies that nurses have a moral and professional commitment to uphold the ideals of compassionate care for all individuals, regardless of their backgrounds or circumstances. The statement reinforces nurses' role in the preservation of human caring, which involves a holistic approach including physical, mental, emotional and social components of wellbeing. This involves working as advocates and protectors of vulnerable groups.

Activity 5.2   Evidence-based practice and research

To address the issue of reducing financial stress on nursing students, you may have chosen any of the options, as all are likely to have some degree of impact. For example, if you choose grass-roots organising, you can band together with others to advocate for policy changes, such as increased financial support for nursing students. This type of activism can build a strong support network through community-driven efforts and create lasting change.

Activity 5.3   Critical thinking

One example of support Bernadette could seek is connecting with professional nursing organisations that promote diversity and inclusion. She may also seek to gain insights into the experiences of others and support available through social media. Her tutor at university is another source of support that may provide ongoing support. Abigail's suggestion that Bernadette speaks with the Student Union may be considered a positive step because it gave Bernadette a way to address the issue and join forces with others who shared her goals. However, a potential con is that it could take time and focus away from her studies. Bernadette shouldn't necessarily be responsible for raising awareness of these important issues – the university and hospital have a duty here.

Activity 5.4   Reflection

Here are a few other ways to promote environmental issues in nursing and healthcare:

- Curriculum Development: Promote the inclusion of environmental sustainability in healthcare into the core curriculum through discussions with your lecturers.
- Support a Sustainable Healthcare Fair to showcase sustainable healthcare products, technology and practices. Invite local healthcare representatives, businesses and innovators.
- Social media campaigns: Promote healthcare sustainability through social media. Create informative posts and online events.

Activity 5.5   Reflection

If you were to draw a mind map with the suggested topic areas, you may have had branches containing information such as the following:

Mental health

- Increase public knowledge and education on mental health in order to minimise stigma.
- Increase accessibility to mental health services.
- Increase mental health support in schools and workplaces.

Environmental equity

- Encourage clean air and water policy in all areas.
- Promote fair access to green places.
- Encourage the use of environmentally friendly practices in healthcare settings.

Social health determinants

- Increase access to high-quality education and employment opportunities.
- Policies that alleviate food and housing insecurity should be supported.
- Advocate for equal access to healthcare.

If you were to look online, you may start by learning more about specific projects or efforts undertaken by nurse activists connected to the topic by exploring various nursing journals, blogs and professional nursing organisation websites.

Activity 5.6   Critical thinking

Opinions vary. Some support the strikes, arguing that nurses, like all workers, should have the right to advocate for better working conditions and fair compensation, especially given their critical role in healthcare. Some worry strikes will disrupt patient care. In terms of public perception, these campaigns could promote nurses' work and garner public support. It can illuminate nurses' difficult working conditions and low pay, despite their vital role in healthcare. If the strikes disrupt patient care, they could be harmful. Nurses may weigh several factors when voting on a strike. If they think their working conditions, pay or benefits are unfair, and negotiations have failed, they may think a strike is the best way to change them. If they think a strike could harm patient care or there are better ways to advocate for change, they might vote against it. Personal finances and job security may affect this decision. It's complicated, so weigh the pros and cons carefully if you have to make this choice.

Further reading

Barr, J and Dowding, L (2022) *Leadership in health care.* London: Sage.

This book focuses on healthcare leadership and management, specifically the role of nurses as leaders and change agents in the healthcare system.

Price, B (2021) *Critical thinking and writing in nursing.* London, Sage.

This book will guide you in the development of critical thinking skills and effective writing.

Useful websites

Royal College of Nursing: **www.rcn.org.uk/**

The world's largest nursing union and professional body, representing and supporting nursing staff across the UK. The website offers resources as well as information on political advocacy and nursing-related campaigns.

Nursing Times: **www.nursingtimes.net/**

The website is a source of nursing news, analysis and opinion. It contains articles on a variety of topics, including healthcare policy, activism and the role of the nursing profession in shaping healthcare delivery.

Chapter 6 Population health

Chapter aims

After reading this chapter, you will be able to:

- define population health;
- explain your role as a nurse in a population health context;
- describe how population health impinges on outcomes experienced by your patient;
- collaboratively plan care with your patient that is holistic and goes beyond the immediate issues of the presenting condition.

Introduction

Have you ever wondered about the future lives of the patients in your care? What will happen to them in not only the days after going home but in the months and years that follow? Will they experience better health or are they destined to continue to experience poor health and face a future where illness and hospitalisations will continue to impinge on their lives?

These are important questions. You would want those in your care to have a future where they live fulfilling lives without illness. From a wider perspective, facilitating healthier lives has benefits for healthcare provision. Encouraging independence and minimising the need for healthcare is beneficial to everyone as individuals and wider society.

These are key concerns in this chapter, where you will be introduced to concepts and ideas from a sub-discipline of the social sciences, namely population health. This subject investigates what determines the health of populations, and hence of individuals. It emphasises the role played by social contexts in largely determining health and disease. Insights from this subject can enable you to better understand your patients and holistically plan care that goes beyond the immediate presenting condition. That has the potential of long-term benefits to those in your care.

What is population health?

Population health is a subject that brings together a range of social sciences to explain health. It is sometimes confused with public health but goes further (Kings Fund, 2022). It is a concern of all health professionals rather than specific to dedicated roles. That means it is of note to all nurses, and so also for you.

More specifically, Kindig and Stoddart (2003) put forward the following widely used definition of population health:

The [health] outcomes of a group of individuals, including the distribution of such outcomes.

Their definition has three parts: (1) that a population is a group of people; (2) the health of these groups, or outcomes, can be measured; and (3) that the health of those groups, or populations, varies. Overall, it gives emphasis to the idea that health is at least as much about communities as about individuals.

> ## Case study: Ellie (part 1)
>
> Ellie is admitted into your care of the medical ward in which you work. She is a 65-year-old woman who has developed community-acquired pneumonia that is proving resistant to
>
> *(Continued)*

treatment. Her treatment follows national guidelines (NICE, 2021) and you work with her to develop nursing care that ensures her activities of living are met. The intention is that she will be discharged back home once her condition has shown signs of responding to treatment and her symptoms have eased.

From your perspective as a nurse, does her social situation make any difference to the care that you provide?

The case study will be picked up on again later in this chapter.

A population is simply a group of people who have attributes in common. Think about Ellie, the woman who forms the basis of the case study in this chapter. She is a woman who lives somewhere in the United Kingdom in the early stages of the twenty-first century. These are only some of the groups to which she can be seen as belonging. You might also consider a range of other aspects to her life, such as her income, housing circumstances, level of education, as well as many others. All of these attributes have implications for her health.

You will see from the quote that Kindig and Stoddart (2003) also refer to outcomes. Some individuals are healthier than others. The same can be considered for populations. You measure individuals' health through, for example, their blood pressure, or if they have long-term conditions. So the same can be done for populations. Various measures are drawn on to summarise population health, such as the incidence and prevalence of disease (Stewart, 2016). Incidence is a measure of how many new cases occur in a population over some time, such as the number of new cases of community-acquired pneumonia over a year. Prevalence is a measure of how many people have a condition at a point in time, say the number of people who have chronic obstructive airways disease per 10,000 people in Scotland.

Another widely used outcome, or indicator of population health, is life expectancy. Life expectancy reflects more than just how long on average people live. It indicates the general health of a population (Sen, 1998). A person who is in good health will likely live longer than another who has poor health. A population with a long average life expectancy will be generally healthier than one where people die younger. Hence life expectancy can also be seen as providing a good summary indication of population health.

Activity 6.1   Critical thinking

Think about yourself as an individual and consider the following questions:

- What are the social groups to which you belong?
- What are the attributes you have in common that makes you part of that group?

Take Ellie's situation in the context of the wider population. Recent figures from the Office for National Statistics (ONS) indicate that the average life expectancy at birth for females in the United Kingdom is 83 years (ONS, 2021). The same source demonstrates that a woman aged 65 years, such as Ellie, might expect to live for another 21 years. These figures are calculated from age-specific mortality rates and describe the average across the population. It is not that Ellie will reach the age of 86 years and suddenly drop dead. It simply provides an indication of the health experienced across the population: in this case women in the UK based on death rates between 2018 and 2020.

What is notable is that figures differ from one population to another. Average life expectancy figures for the UK are not as high as people living in some other countries. A recent report from the United Nations Development Programme (UNDP, 2022) indicated the population of the UK lives almost four years on average less than those in Switzerland. Conversely, and as indicated in that report, life expectancy in the UK is markedly higher than in many other countries. So the country in which Ellie lives has implications for her health.

As Kindig and Stoddart's quote indicates, health can also vary *within* populations. Again, drawing on life expectancy as an indicator, between 2017 and 2019, people living in the most deprived areas of the United Kingdom had on average shorter lives than those in the least deprived (The Health Foundation, 2022). In England, life expectancy in the most deprived areas for men was more than nine years shorter than for those in the least deprived. The same was true within Scotland and Wales. The UK is not unique in that variation. Similar findings have been demonstrated internationally (Mackenbach et al., 2008). The part of the country where Ellie lives will therefore also have implications for her health.

Just why groups of people have different levels of health is complex. It is not reasonable to suppose that these are just the results of random chance differences: the population of the United Kingdom is over 60 million people. What research has demonstrated is that these differences result from the circumstances in which people live: social determinants. These will be considered next.

The social determinants of health

Health is often seen as a combination of a person's own decision-making and luck. They can choose behaviours that are conducive to good health or not. And whether they get a disease or not is largely down to chance. Such understandings though cannot explain the shared experiences of health discussed in the previous section.

Population health challenges such notions. This is not to say that individual decisions or luck do not have a role. Smoking, for example, has been demonstrated to increase the risk of developing community-acquired pneumonia (Almirall et al., 2017). However, health is shaped in large part by circumstances into which they are born, and through their life course. It is these circumstances, shared by others in the same social and economic groups, that largely shape health.

Figure 6.1 provides a graphical indication of these social determinants. It highlights that overarching everything else, it is living conditions that are most influential in determining health outcomes. These situations will affect whole populations, and hence the differences that can be seen between different groups. They include a range of social aspects that will be shared by many, such as the level of education, water and sanitation, and housing. Note that healthcare services are included among these higher-level determinants, though it is only one across a number. Healthcare provision alone is not a cure-all for poor health outcomes experienced by populations.

Also of note is that individual lifestyle factors are a component that contributes towards outcomes. The overarching social determinants also influence the degree to which people will engage in those elements. Poor health behaviours are thus themselves socially determined. Decisions made by individuals regarding smoking, alcohol consumption or exercise are influenced by social factors.

That Ellie is in hospital with a chest infection is thus very likely more than a chance occurrence. It may be that her social circumstances have led her to experience poor health which, either directly or indirectly, have resulted in her illness and hospitalisation.

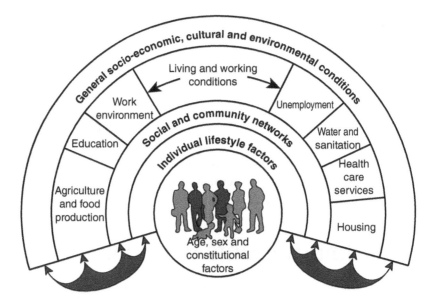

Figure 6.1　The Dahlgren and Whitehead model of health determinants

Source: Dahlgren and Whitehead (1993), cited in Dahlgreen and Whitehead (2021)

There is a range of reasons why these determinants are so influential to health. Each of the overarching determinants indicated in Figure 6.1 will be linked to outcomes through their specific causal pathways. They are also interlinked and often accentuate the effect of one another. People with fewer educational opportunities while growing up are more likely to experience unemployment and low income. Those with low income are going to be more likely to have substandard housing. And so on.

Student voices: Carol

If you don't have a job, you don't feel your worth in society.

Carol, 2nd Year Adult Student Nurse

Activity 6.2   Reflection

Do you agree with Carol, the subject of the scenario?

What impact do you think this may have on the health prospects of unemployed people? Why does this matter to you in your nursing role?

An outline answer is given at the end of the chapter.

As has already been alluded to, healthcare can also be seen as a social determinant. That would be so where people had to pay for healthcare. However, even where access is free, use can still be socially determined. What is referred to as the *inverse care law* suggests that those with the most need (in other words those in socially marginalised circumstances who experience the worst health) are also the least likely to access the services and support they need (Marmot, 2018). This is important in thinking through your role as a nurse.

Take for example breast cancer screening services. Evidence internationally shows that uptake is lower for people from deprived communities (Smith et al., 2019). One outcome is likely to be that where cancer does develop then help will be sought at a later point with adverse implications for health.

Reasons why the inverse care law can result even in the context of openly available services are complex and often work through the other determinants of health. Take education as an example. Poor literacy may make it more difficult to understand health education messages or information provided on posters or leaflets. That will clearly impinge on health behaviours but may also make using screening services less likely. Likewise other healthcare provisions.

As a nursing student, you are likely to have found a lot of the language related to your studies challenging to comprehend. Imagine how difficult it is for someone with poor literacy and for whom health is not the subject of day-to-day discussion or work. Education might also impinge on the confidence needed to speak up and ask questions. Consider what it is like for you to talk to senior staff as a nursing student: not easy. Then put yourself in the place of someone who has rarely been in a healthcare setting, and who might feel self-conscious as to their language.

That self-confidence might be further undermined by a sense of personal blame. People often put their health down to decisions they have made (Blaxter, 1997). Again, that sense of personal blame might reduce self-confidence and ability to ask questions or challenge decisions around their care.

There may be hidden costs to engaging with healthcare services even when access is ostensibly free. Getting to a family doctor might involve a bus journey, itself not easy if in poor health. The fare required might not be easy to find if a person is on a low income, worried about debt and has a list of bills outstanding. It may require taking time off work. The scope for doing so might be limited and may involve a loss of income.

Think back to Ellie's case study. You will remember that she has been diagnosed with community-acquired pneumonia and treatment has commenced. Without knowledge and recognition of the wider determinants of health, her care might go no further than medical treatment. She may have advice around health behaviours, especially if she engages in smoking. With that advice and treatment her breathlessness will hopefully ease, oral antibiotics will be started, and her discharge home will follow. You have done your job.

Yet as a nursing professional, and when recognising the implications of wider determinants of health, there is more that needs to be considered.

Scenario: Catherine

As a recently qualified nurse, you are working with Catherine, a patient on a rehabilitation ward. She experienced a cerebral vascular accident (a stroke) some three weeks earlier which left her with a hemiparesis. An initial assessment, done on admission, highlighted various implications across her activities of daily living, including mobilisation, communication, and eating and drinking. A care plan was put in place in consultation and involving the multidisciplinary team including nursing staff, speech therapist, physiotherapist and occupational therapist. Since then, she has made excellent progress and is managing her activities of living largely independently. Mobilising continues to be challenging, though even there she is making good progress with a walking aid. You are putting plans in place for her discharge.

> ## Activity 6.3   Leadership and management
>
> While working with Catherine on her discharge plan, what are the population health issues you might want to discuss with her?
>
> Think carefully about Catherine's social circumstances: income; housing; social networks and so forth.
>
> *An outline answer is given at the end of the chapter.*

The nursing role in relation to the social determinants of health

As a nursing professional, you need to go further than just addressing the immediate, the obvious, and the here and now. The ideal is to work 'upstream' and prevent problems from occurring in the first place. The upstream metaphor is that rather than just constantly pulling people out of a river who are drowning, you look to see why they are falling in to begin with and take preventative actions (Kuehnert et al., 2022). That ultimately means addressing the social determinants themselves and so addressing the injustice that results from the circumstances into which people are born. The chapter on activism shows how you, as a nurse, can contribute to that endeavour. In this chapter, we will focus on what you can do as an intrinsic part of your nursing care.

The Institute for Health Equality (2013) suggested ways in which healthcare professionals can effectively contribute to addressing social inequalities. Two key elements are (1) through learning and teaching about the determinants of health, and (2) through engaging with individuals and their communities.

Learning and teaching

By reading this book, you are living the first of those steps. You are raising your awareness of health and healthcare, social determinants, and the role that you play. Understanding how social circumstances influence the health of populations, and hence of the individuals that make up those populations, places you in a position to better develop care and activities to make a difference.

In the not-too-distant future, you will become a registered nurse. Once you are on the register, an important part of your role will be as a clinical supervisor. That places you in a position to support the learning of future registrants and hence to raise their awareness of social determinants, how they influence health and the implications for care. The opportunities to develop learning will contribute to a more empathetic healthcare system better able to support the needs of its patients regardless of social background.

You are encouraged in your learning to think critically. One neat way to do this is to think about your subjects considering the social determinants of health. When in tutorials, challenge your lecturers as to the implications of population health for the subject they are teaching. Or discuss scenarios in essays that engage with people living lives in different social contexts.

Think about, for example, how you might apply learning around communication to situations where dealing with people with lower levels of literacy. Consider how you might enable open discussion around a diagnosis or treatment. That same critical approach might be applied to any number of subjects you encounter. Think about discharge planning where people live in substandard housing, perhaps that they rent, and where they are limited in alterations that can be made.

The key point is to critically apply the social determinants of health to your learning. No two patients have the same life-course experiences. They all have their own specific set of social circumstances that will have implications for their health and engagement with healthcare services. Applying that thinking to your learning, and to that of those students with whom you work now and in the future, will both develop you and them as more rounded healthcare professionals who can make a difference.

Activity 6.4   Reflection

A comment you might come across is that there is not sufficient time to concern yourself with social issues, such as patients' housing situations or their low income.

How would you respond to colleagues who might suggest that time spent on the wider determinants of health is something that nurses can ill afford?

An outline answer is given at the end of the chapter.

Individuals and communities

Much of what has been said regarding education links in to care provision. The Institute of Health Equity (2013) highlight that an important step towards professionals' contributions towards tackling inequalities is through enabling those in their care to have greater control over their own lives.

Doing so requires the development of trusting relationships where patients feel able to openly share information and concerns. Only through recognising the realities of daily life can you take any steps. Only through sharing information can truly individualised care, care that recognises social circumstances and their implications, be factored into care planning.

Social determinants, as has been touched on in the discussion relating to Figure 6.1, impinge on health-related behaviours. Patient education that is free of blame and more empathetic can enable them to make informed decisions about their lives. It can also enable discussion of the barriers a person has or envisages experiencing in, say, trying to give up smoking. Those two-way discussions can then enable practical thinking as to how these might be overcome. Keep in mind the role of education, and the implications that having had fewer educational opportunities might have for your patient. Especially important is using accessible language and asking patients to repeat back what they have understood. Patience and time are key.

Activity 6.5   Critical thinking

You have been asked to write an essay as a part of a module's assessment. The essay focuses on care of a particular condition – it might be focused on mental health, care of children, a learning difficulty issue or a medical condition. The requirements of the essay include a demonstration of critical thinking. How might a population health angle assist you to meet this aspect?

An outline answer is given at the end of the chapter.

Care planning needs to be a shared endeavour, especially when looking forward to discharge and your patient's life after they have left your care, whether you are in a community or hospital setting. That care planning will require information, and information sharing is an important component of your making a difference to lives in the context of social determinants.

Ascertaining information may also involve taking a social history (Institute of Health Equity, 2013). Various social determinant screening tools have been developed (Andermann, 2018). Whether a social history is taken, or a more formal screening tool is used, the important point is that you will be better placed to act if you have information about social circumstances.

There is no point in gathering information unless you can act. Steps you might take will depend on the specifics of your patient and their situation. That might require referring to agencies better placed to provide support. It may also enable you to tailor care plans better to their needs. Many of the implications of social determinants are going to be beyond what you can do as an individual practitioner, but there are a wealth of other professionals and organisations from whom you might draw regarding each of the social determinants. These might include colleagues from within the NHS or local authorities, such as occupational therapists or social workers. Or it may be through drawing on the many organisations from the voluntary sector that exist to provide advice and support around housing, debt, domestic violence or otherwise.

A key point is that these issues – housing, debt, the experience of violence and so on – will very likely be a considerable anxiety to your patient with serious health implications of their own in the months and years ahead. That is not to negate the presenting condition, which of course must be addressed with urgency. Rather, it is the need for your care to be holistic, and to go beyond the here and now. Your openly engaging with these issues may make more difference in the long-term improvement of their lives. It may avoid future illness and so make a small but important contribution to addressing health inequalities.

Consider again the case study with which this chapter opened. This was a straightforward case of a woman admitted to your care with community-acquired pneumonia. The expectation is that the antibiotics will sort out her problems. Yet that is to treat the case without considering the wider determinants.

Case study: Ellie (part 2)

In the first part of this case study, you learned about Ellie, a patient you are admitting with community-acquired pneumonia. You take a social history and learn that Ellie is living in very poor housing where damp is an issue. She has a long history of homelessness and of financial difficulties. She is concerned as to her employment situation to which being admitted to hospital is not helping. She admits to having been struggling with both physical and mental health for a very long period. She has had numerous chest infections recently but rarely contacted her GP.

As you can ascertain from the second part of her case study, Ellie's situation is more complex than was initially suggested. It is a summary and, of course, there may be very many other issues involved. Even with the information provided, discharging her home without taking into account the social determinants of health is a missed opportunity. Her going home to her current housing circumstances is likely to lead to further health problems and hospitalisations.

Ellie's housing situation is clearly concerning. It has implications for her health both physically and psychologically. This is only one example of housing that has implications for wellbeing. The ETHOS (European Typology of Homelessness and Housing Exclusion) typology of housing lists a range of adverse situations that effectively make people homeless: living in shelters, in fear of violence, have insecure tenure (so under constant threat of eviction), in overcrowded accommodation and so forth (FEANTSA, 2017). Homelessness is much more than rooflessness, with adverse implications for health and hence for holistic care planning.

The point of the case study is to demonstrate how seemingly straightforward care situations may both hide and be the result of underlying social issues. These may in themselves be a cause of the condition that led to admission. It may be that these are of considerable concern to the person involved, and every bit as pressing in the longer term as the more immediate illness.

Solutions are not straightforward. However, having awareness opens the potential for action. This is where drawing on the knowledge and expertise of others is invaluable.

Interprofessional practice is a key strategy. You might discuss with Ellie a referral to the social work team. You could liaise with others to make connections with third-sector organisations in her community who might be able to help, whether regarding her housing, work or financial situation.

Activity 6.6   Critical thinking

What organisations exist in your local area who can provide support to people experiencing challenging social situations?

You might consider the following issues (but don't feel limited to them):

- debt advice;
- benefits;
- legal advice;
- housing and homelessness issues;
- mental health support;
- addiction.

How might these organisations be of help to patients in your care?

An outline answer is given at the end of the chapter.

Holistic care is important. That Ellie has indicated struggling with her mental health might alert you to the very real possibility that she is experiencing depression, something for which you might screen. Treating depression without engaging with the wider determinants is likely to be limited. That said, Ellie is more likely to be able to engage with support if her health is holistically considered. Both are important.

An empathetic approach to health education and sharing information might open new ideas for Ellie. The case study does not touch on things such as her diet, exercise or smoking. These may be less of a concern to her at that point. Recognising social context and openly discussing may enable Ellie to make changes that will benefit her health sometime in the future.

A therapeutic relationship is key to recognising the realities of life after discharge from your care, and to thinking through how they might be supported to overcome those social and economic barriers to health and healthcare. The same goes for all patients regardless of social background but is especially beneficial where deprivation might act as a barrier to fulfilling care. As indicated earlier in the chapter, a key element of the inverse care law is that people may feel less confident in speaking up for themselves. Avoiding medical jargon and giving opportunities and encouraging questions might better enable you to understand needs and advocate on their behalf if necessary.

Chapter summary

This chapter has considered how population health can have relevance to your patients, their health and healthcare. The social determinants of health make more likely that some groups are more likely to experience ill health than others and can make engagement with services more difficult even if when free at the point of delivery.

Ellie's case study has illustrated how apparently straightforward cases can have underlying issues that should be of concern to you as a nurse. There are a multitude of housing situations that might be considered as homelessness, from the obvious – rooflessness – to less obvious but nonetheless concerning, such as Ellie and her damp housing. And that is only to consider one of the social determinants of health: housing. Factor in all the others touched on in Figure 6.1 and your population health role becomes ever more apparent. Add in that those most impacted by the social determinants of health are the most likely to develop poor health and so come into your care.

Further, the condition chosen for the case study was for illustrative purposes. Any might have been chosen. It is not only physiological conditions for which population health has implications. Mental health is also very much underpinned by social determinants. Homelessness, poverty, unemployment and so forth create long-term stress and so will act as an underlying cause of issues such as depression. Her age was also illustrative only. The issues addressed by population health are just as applicable to families and children, and people with learning difficulties. Regardless of your field of nursing, the issues discussed in this chapter apply to your care planning and provision.

The focus has also been very much on how you can support patients who have come into your care. Thinking upstream – how to prevent the social injustices of social determinants – is important. Preventing problems from happening is always going to be preferable, and it is to that issue that the chapter on activism is focused. You will inevitably meet patients whose lives have been damaged as a result of circumstances they did not choose. Endeavouring to ensure that their future holds more promise is a valuable contribution your nursing care can make.

Activities: Brief outline answers

Activity 6.1   Critical thinking

There are many dimensions to your identity you might have indicated here. These may relate to social or geographical aspects of your life. Geographically, you might have considered where you are from or live. Or you might have considered social aspects of your identity, perhaps your age, gender or your occupation, perhaps being a nurse or a student. These are only examples. Every person will have multiple social identities that interact with one another.

Figure 6.1 is especially helpful for thinking through how these different aspects of your identity might have implications for your health. As you will have read through the course of this chapter (and in the book more generally), the social world can impact on your health in many ways: physically, say through pollution or exposure to infectious diseases; or indirectly, through psychosocial stress or understanding of health-related behaviours. They interact with each other, for example level of education having implications for employment and occupation, and so also for income and housing. Implications for these different dimensions will also be influenced by age and gender, as well as health status itself.

Activity 6.2   Reflection

As was shown in Figure 6.1, employment is an important determinant of health. Vancea and Utzet (2017) provide a scoping study of the impact of both unemployment and tenuous employment on the health of younger people. Note that mental health problems are especially common among people in such situations. There are a range of reasons why that would be, but these could all link into feelings of self-worth. Employment is for many people an important part of their identity. You may well take pride in considering yourself to be a nurse, for example. Occupation also links into other determinants such as income and housing, both of which have important links to both identity and health outcomes.

Treating patients as people is key so that they feel able to share concerns such as around their employment situation, and attendant issues such as financial or housing problems. Nursing care has a role both for the immediate health of patients but also for the longer term. You can enable links between patients and organisations that might be able to advise. Interdisciplinary practice is valuable and reaching out beyond healthcare professions of considerable help. In the case of people experiencing unemployment, there may be financial or housing issues to which you might point people or enable links through your social services colleagues.

Activity 6.3   Leadership and management

A key insight from population health is the importance of social and geographic context. In the short term, ensuring Catherine can manage her activities of daily living is clearly key. Catherine's social circumstances could have implications, particularly regarding mobility. Given her mobility issues, stairs might present a problem. Scope for changes to facilitate may be influenced by the type of housing in which she resides.

Understanding the situation at an early stage is important and liaising closely with social work or occupational health colleagues of considerable value. So often where population health and nursing are concerned, interprofessional working is central. In the scenario, these colleagues have clearly been involved from an early stage (which is excellent). Discussing these issues with them and with Catherine will help elucidate the situation and identify ways forward.

You can also consider the wider determinants with a view to supporting Catherine's long-term health. Having a stroke may have implications for her ability to continue working, and hence also for her income and housing tenure. Again, thinking socially and being aware of opportunities to link to other agencies can make a considerable difference now and even more so for the future. You might also consider Catherine's health-related behaviours. She may or may not have been at higher risk of experiencing a stroke because of, for example, smoking, diet or otherwise.

Minimise the possibility of recurrence and explore with her opportunities for change, such as stopping smoking or changing diet (see Linsley and Roll, 2023).

Activity 6.4 Reflection

This is a very challenging question that you may have been considering or might come across in practice. There's no doubting that health services are very stretched and inevitably that has implications for nursing practice. You will have to prioritise when planning care day to day. Yet that does not mean that population health cannot be a central part of your holistic care.

For a start, just being aware of how social determinants impinge on people's lives will assist you in prioritising more effectively. Further, many of the steps you might take are not in themselves very time consuming yet can make a marked difference both in the short and long term. Anxieties around housing or money induce stress which harms quality of life. Whether through referral or simply raising awareness of available support, nurses can make a difference beyond what would be achieved by focus on a medical model.

Activity 6.5 Critical thinking

You will often be asked to demonstrate critical thinking in an assessment, whether an essay or a presentation. One way you might do this is by thinking about population health. Regardless of what the topic of focus might be, social determinants will have implications. They impinge on health (and hence even the need for healthcare), for the ability of people to engage and utilise healthcare services, and for their lives both while in your care and afterwards. Look back at essay questions you have already answered and think about the different angles that could have been taken if you had considered housing, deprivation, poverty and so on. You might think through how a situation will differ depending on if someone is housed or homeless, younger or older, employed or unemployed. The list is endless but will demonstrate thinking that recognises the diversity of people's lives and what that means for person-centred and holistic nursing care planning.

Activity 6.6 Critical thinking

Answers to this question will differ depending on where you are in the country. Some support services are national though many are run more locally. Good starting points are to talk with lecturers or clinical supervisors. They may have different insights depending on their own area of expertise. You might also look at the pages of Citizens Advice (www.citizensadvice.org.uk/). It has up-to-date advice as well as being a useful resource for people experiencing problems with housing, income and many other issues. You might also find the web pages of your local council helpful. They will very often if not always have a search facility. If you enter a search term such as 'homelessness' you will find information directly relating to the council, but also to other sources of help, which can include organisations whose remit and expertise is helping people in such situations.

Further reading

Cohen N and Galea S (2011) *Population mental health.* Abingdon: Routledge.

This book has a United States focus but provides a good overview of population mental health. It provides a good insight into how the social determinants of health are every bit as applicable to mental health issues as they are to physiological illness.

Institute of Health Equity (2013) *Working for health equity: the role of health care professionals.* London: Institute of Health Equity. www.instituteofhealthequity.org/resources-reports/working-for-health-equity-the-role-of-health-professionals/working-for-health-equity-the-role-of-health-professionals-full-report.pdf [last accessed 4 April 2023]

This report has some discussion of the role healthcare professionals can play in making a difference at a population level.

Marmot M (2016) *The health gap: improving health in an unequal world.* London: Bloomsbury.

An accessible book that explains how social hierarchy impacts on health and implications for approaches to wellbeing.

Useful websites

The Health Foundation: **www.health.org.uk/publications**

This provides reports that touch on the wider determinants of health and implications for healthcare. Their web page provides a portal that can develop your understanding of social issues and encourage your epidemiological imagination with all the resulting links to your nursing care practice.

The Institute of Health Equity: **www.instituteofhealthequity.org/home**

This raises awareness of the social determinants of health and advocates for policies to address them. On their website you will find a range of materials that aim to support work towards a fairer society including papers reporting evidence around impacts of issues such as COVID-19 and its implications for health equity.

The Glasgow Centre for Population Health: **www.gcph.co.uk/**

This focuses on poverty in Scotland and its impact on health, but information is applicable to policy and practice much more widely. You will find a range of topics covered from children and families, through health behaviours, communities and population trends, through to financial issues – a very valuable resource for developing your understanding and thinking around the social determinants of health and implications for your practice.

The King's Fund: **www.kingsfund.org.uk/publications/population-health-approach**

The King's Fund provides information on population health and its implications for healthcare. Their resources provide a very helpful overview of the subject including associated policy at national and local levels.

Chapter 7 Social science research methods

Chapter aims

After reading this chapter, you will be able to:

- explain the value of understanding social science research methods to nursing professionals in practice, advocacy and education;
- discuss major approaches to research used to answer questions in the social sciences;
- describe sources of information on the social sciences;
- consider the ethical issues that apply to research in the social sciences.

Introduction

This book has to this point explained the value of the social sciences to you in your role as a nurse. Underlying ideas have been drawn from a considerable literature reporting on research that covers the breadth of health and healthcare. Ideas drawn from them have then been used to explain ways in which they apply to you, as a nursing student, and with a view to your future career.

As with any area of your practice, you cannot just accept what you are told or have read. The source makes no difference, even if it is the most reputable of sources (yes, even this book!). The NMC expects that nurses should understand research and to think critically. There are good reasons for them doing so. Claims can be made that, when investigated in more detail, turn out to be founded on poor (or even no) evidence. So, whenever you hear a claim, you need to question, question, question.

This chapter provides an overview of how evidence is developed in the social sciences. It starts by discussing the value of going further than accepting claims at face value. That makes the case for investing time into learning about the methods used by social scientists and appreciating the logic used. The next section provides a brief overview of the two main approaches to social science research: quantitative and qualitative. Inevitably this can be no more than an introduction. Deepening understanding will require you to go further. It is to how you might do so that the chapter moves, then moves with the intention of enthusing you to develop your understanding of the social sciences on into the rest of your career. To start with, consider in more detail the value of going behind claims and developing an understanding of the research.

Activity 7.1 Leadership and management

Imagine that in the future you have been promoted into a leadership position within an acute mental health unit. During your time on the unit, you have noticed that the transitional period immediately after admission to the unit can be challenging for some individuals. You believe that changes to the admission process would be beneficial and decide to begin introducing these and to evaluate their effectiveness.

Think about why you might you wish to take into account the following elements in your evaluation:

- housing status on admission;
- employment status on admission;
- ethnicity;
- place of residence.

An outline answer is given at the end of this chapter.

Recognising the value of research to you and your practice

The introduction has already pointed towards a key reason as to why understanding research is so important. You cannot simply accept claims you hear being made. That is only one reason though why understanding evidence that underpins claims is so valuable to you as a nursing student.

An important starting point is that understanding research can be enriching to you personally. Researchers draw on methods that have a logic to how they ascertain answers to the questions they pose. You can find your passion for the social sciences ignited when you read about the ingenious approaches that have elucidated evidence on which understanding of the social world is based.

That resulting passion can enthuse you to deepen your knowledge of the social sciences to the benefit of you personally and your patients. It can build your confidence to act as advocate, whether for a patient in your care or when liaising with colleagues in management or with policymakers.

You might also find that the resulting enthusiasm will encourage you to take forward your own research. That might lead you to take courses in the social sciences that involve a research element. Or you might use what you learn when you are involved in practice evaluation. The quote provided in the following Student Voices box highlights the potential of clinical research to influencing nursing practice. The same applies to taking forward social sciences research. As you have read in this book so far, social circumstances have considerable implications for people's lives, and hence for how they engage with your care. Factoring that into how you evaluate practice can enable these powerful influences on your patients' lives to be recognised and considered.

Student voices: From Grønning et al., 2022, page 5

In the following passage, a student nurse shares their experience of undertaking a clinical research project during the latter stages of their studies:

We are able to contribute to changes as a result of our project, and it will influence our work as future nurses.

Scenario: Jo

Jo is a student nurse on placement. She has impressive in-depth knowledge of medical conditions she is encountering in clinical areas. You have previously discussed with Jo the social sciences and considered implications for patient care. Jo though is sceptical that it really matters. Surely, we should just focus on presenting illnesses, she opines.

This gets you thinking. You recognised that Jo is demonstrating professionalism in not just accepting claims. So how do we know that the social context within which people's lives are lived influences their health and their engagement with health services? What is the evidence?

Activity 7.2   Reflection

You are going to be a registered nurse after graduating and will be involved in supervising and assessing students such as Jo. It can be difficult for students to appreciate their role beyond addressing presenting medical or psychiatric conditions. As the above scenario indicates, this scepticism is both healthy and professional.

How might you use research to convince Jo that understanding social dimensions and their implications is important? What are the key points you might make and what might you do to facilitate her learning?

An outline answer is given at the end of this chapter.

How is research done in the social sciences?

You might have come across health research in your studies to date. The two research areas – health and social sciences – share much with one another. As you will have read in earlier chapters, health is largely socially determined. So, understanding how and why will require approaches not so different from those developed for health research. You will find systematic reviews, randomised controlled trials and qualitative studies as much in the social as health sciences. Social scientists must consider the same kinds of issues as found in the health sciences, especially around ethics and governance.

Ethics

Informed consent is every bit as important in the social sciences as in health research. This requires that participants are informed as to the purpose of their involvement in a study and given opportunity to decide if they wish to take part. As in health research, and healthcare, confidentiality is important and, as long as the researchers have no reason to believe the participant or wider public is in danger, nothing should be disclosed that would enable the individual to be identified.

The researchers must submit their research proposal to an ethics committee and explain what will be involved. They must outline potential issues and the steps that will be taken to mitigate them, for example, the information that will be given to potential participants to ensure that consent is informed.

Ethics committees comprise other academics and lay members of the public. They will consider the proposed research and will often require the research team make changes to ensure the study meets high ethical standards. Only once they are content with what is proposed will the research be approved and allowed to proceed.

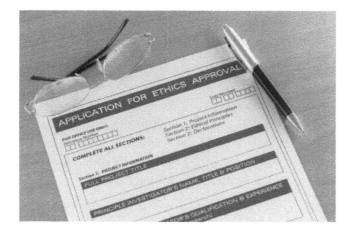

Figure 7.1 A research ethics application form

Source: iStock.com/Pixsooz

Methods

Researchers look to use methods that will enable research questions to be answered so that findings can be trusted. These will often be set out in a protocol before the study commences. Methods are identified that will convincingly enable answers to be achieved. When they come to report their findings in journal papers, their research will be scrutinised by experts in their field, an approach called 'peer review' (see the following Concept Summary). They have to convince their colleagues that methods chosen can convincingly answer the questions.

Concept summary: Peer review

Peer review of social science research involves a quality check by experts in the same field. It involves experienced researchers, or 'peers', in the same field or discipline evaluating research papers or proposals. Peers critically evaluate the research for accuracy, validity and reliability to ensure that its methods, analysis and conclusions are ethical and advance that field of knowledge. This process ensures the credibility and quality of academic journals, books and grant proposals. Peer review in social science research can also assess cultural sensitivity and ethical consideration for the groups studied. In evidence-based practice, nursing students may encounter peer-reviewed sources. Peer-reviewed sources ensure that your practice is based on scientifically sound information.

Broadly there are two groups of research: quantitative and qualitative. Systematic reviews form another approach, though these endeavour to bring together evidence from other studies. Under the umbrella of each of these broad methodological approaches are sub-groups. Quantitative methods are widely used by researchers including demographers, social epidemiologists and psychologists. Qualitative methods are central to social anthropology and widely used in sociology.

The relative value of different approaches is the subject of considerable debate. You will over time develop your own views informed by your reading, discussions and reflection. The view taken in this book is that each approach is valuable for answering specific kinds of questions. Some research draws on more than one method including both quantitative and qualitative, each providing different insights into the issue or issues of interest (McKendrick, 1999; 2020). So both quantitative and qualitative methods are valuable and worth understanding.

Quantitative approaches in the social sciences

Quantitative methods are, as the name implies, used to quantify. That enables researchers to describe groups of people, be they residents of a geographical area, patients admitted to a hospital, or otherwise. For example, demographers can describe the age distribution of different populations, important for planning. Epidemiologists can estimate the prevalence of different diseases, with value to considering healthcare provision. Both have clear implications for planning service provision. This is only a start of the value of quantitative methods. They can also be used to ask questions to understand what the effects of social circumstances or policy interventions are for people's lives.

Various approaches can be used. Randomised controlled trials (RCTs) are less common in the social sciences compared to health. These are studies that randomly assign people to a 'treatment group' or a 'control group'. The treatment group receives the intervention while the control group usually has the standards approach. Outcomes of interest are then compared one to the other to assess if there are differences. One example of an RCT is provided in the next Research Summary box.

Research summary: 'housing first' approaches to addressing homelessness

A Canadian study reported by Aubry et al. (2015) randomly assigned homeless people who had severe mental health problems to two different housing programmes. The researchers

(Continued)

then assessed the extent to which one or the other better enabled people to maintain their tenancy and whether it made any difference to their wellbeing.

In brief, the 'intervention group' had housing prioritised, an approach called 'housing first'. Those randomly allocated to this group received a tenancy that was not dependent on them engaging with health services. The 'control group' received what was the standard approach to supporting people in situations of homelessness, which included various support and outreach services. The sample sizes were large, with over 900 people taking part in the study.

A year later, the researchers reported that those receiving 'housing first' were more likely to be stably housed and had a higher quality of life. The study provides strong evidence that people who are in situations of homelessness and who have severe mental health problems, if given the opportunity, are very able to maintain a tenancy and, further, will have better outcomes as a result.

This study (and others like it) provide convincing evidence that housing can and should be a priority in supporting people to moving out of homelessness even if they are experiencing mental health problems. The study design, an RCT, makes for particularly convincing evidence. Being able to explain that evidence can be a powerful means of advocacy.

Activity 7.3   Evidence-based practice and research

What are the implications of the above study from the point of view of nursing care?

Given the research was done in Canada, do you think that the findings would apply when supporting people who are homeless in the United Kingdom?

An outline answer is given at the end of this chapter.

More common than RCTs in the social sciences are observational studies. These studies use data from very large-scale surveys, sometimes involving many thousands of people, and that have information at different points in time (longitudinal data). Researchers can also use data from sources such as the census, a questionnaire that ascertains information about everyone living in the UK every ten years, and data routinely collected by organisations as part of their service provision, such as from cancer screening or hospitalisations. Analysis of data such as this enables insights about populations at a point in time, and to ascertain outcomes that result sometime after (see the following Research Summary for an example).

Observational studies are often more practical and ethical than RCTs. They do not require the researchers to 'intervene' in any way. As the name of the approach suggests, they observe what happens. The data already exists for large numbers of people and going back in time. That enables timely analysis of outcomes that occur many years later.

Research summary: Implications of deprivation for survival after cancer diagnosis

A study reported by Ingleby et al. (2022) investigated the implications of deprivation for patients diagnosed with cancer. They used an anonymised representative sample of people drawn from the census who had been diagnosed with colorectal, prostate or breast cancer. Cancer diagnosis was ascertained using cancer registration data. They then compared how long people survived after diagnosis and the extent to which this differed by deprivation.

Findings demonstrated that an individual's social situation, indicated by income, education or occupation, had a marked effect on survival. They also found that where people lived mattered. Even considering individual circumstances, living in more deprived areas meant, on average, shorter lives after cancer diagnosis.

The study provides indication that social circumstances impact on life chances after being diagnosed with cancer. They also indicated that where people live also matters.

Activity 7.4   Evidence-based practice and research

Consider the observational study described in the previous Research Summary.

What might be the implications for you if working in cancer care?

An outline answer is given at the end of this chapter.

Analysis of quantitative data

Studies using quantitative methods use statistical approaches. These might seem quite off-putting when you first look at papers, but they have some basic underlying concepts that are intuitive. The question posed is whether differences between groups might be just a chance finding, or whether the gap is so great that it is more likely to be the result of something underlying, such as the level of deprivation experienced (see the previous Research Summary). The bigger the gap, the less likely the result happened by chance and especially if there are large numbers of people in the analysis (hence quantitative studies generally have sample sizes). Where that happens, the researchers will also estimate the effect size, which is an indication as to the degree to which the relationship in question matters.

That is, of course, a very brief description of how statistical approaches work. There are a multitude of approaches used by quantitative researchers, but that basic principle underpins most of the approaches used. Grasp these underlying principles and you will understand much of the work done using quantitative methods. At the end of this chapter you will find other books that can help you come to understand in statistics in greater depth. The key message is that statistics are, with a little study, accessible. Dip into papers and try not to be put off by what initially appear to be obscure numbers.

In short, quantitative methods are a means by which long-term outcomes can be studied and ascertained. The ability to measure and assess them comes from statistics. They can provide compelling evidence that is sometimes surprising – challenging our assumptions and enthusing your practice.

Qualitative methods

Qualitative methods include approaches used to explore, understand and interpret social phenomena, human behaviour and experiences. They often focus on the meanings that people attach to issues that impact their lives. Qualitative methods attempt to understand each individual's perspective and account for their unique context. In doing so it aims to provide rich, detailed and in-depth insights into the subject under inquiry. Creswell and Poth (2018) identify five qualitative research methodologies: phenomenology, ethnography, narrative research, case study research and grounded theory (see the Concept Summary).

Developing a deeper understanding of the challenges your patients face can be furthered through reading and learning about qualitative methods. These approaches generally have far smaller samples than quantitative with the intention of achieving greater depth and nuance.

Various approaches are used by qualitative researchers. Examples of these are shown in the following Concept Summary.

Concept summary: Qualitative research methods

Ethnography: Also known as participant observation. It has its roots in the discipline of social anthropology. The researcher endeavours to embed themselves in a particular social setting, which might be anything from a community to a hospital ward. They then immerse themselves in what is happening, collecting data through observations, interviews, reading documents and so on. Their intention is to understand people's lives in the context of their social setting.

Grounded Theory: uses an inductive methodology that entails systematic data collection and analysis in order to develop a 'grounded' theoretical framework. If you were to use this approach in the future it would help you to generate theory based on empirical data, which can then be used to develop effective nursing interventions.

Narrative Research: A method for comprehending and interpreting people's stories in order to gain insights into human experiences. You could use narrative research to appreciate patients' lived experiences, thereby improving patient-centred care.

Phenomenology: A method for investigating people's lived experiences and the meanings they assign to those experiences. Phenomenological research is a method for gaining a deeper understanding of patients' perceptions, feelings and experiences with illness or healthcare, resulting in more empathetic and holistic care.

Data for qualitative research comes from a variety of sources but very often through interviews. These can be anything from structured interviews, where participants are all asked the same questions and in the same order, through to semi-structured interviews where the interaction is much closer to a conversation. Effective qualitative interviewing is a craft that takes practice to master (Brinkmann and Kvale, 2015). It involves active listening, empathy, rapport-building, sensitivity and adaptability, while maintaining a neutral and unbiased approach. Data is captured in the form of words, rather than the numeric or categorical data of the quantitative researcher. Interviews are usually captured using a digital recorder and then typed up verbatim and often in considerable detail, including not only words used but also observations. McGrath, Palmgren and Liljedahl (2019) explain that this process enables the researcher to gain a deeper understanding of information the person has shared.

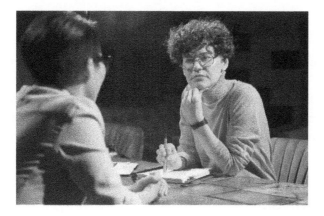

Figure 7.2 A social science researcher interviews a participant

Source: iStock.com/SeventyFour

Interviews can be held in an office or someone's home. Or they might be done while walking with the interviewer. Each approach has its own benefits. For example, a walking interview might enable a person to relax more and enable insights that would be lost if sat down and focusing (Kinney, 2017). Or it might provide a basis for discussing the area in which they live or work. The key point is that the methods used enable different insights.

Another widely used qualitative approach is to use focus groups. These involve participants being asked questions as small groups. Doing so is likely to elicit different insights than if participants were asked the same questions. They can hear what others are saying, which might trigger thinking that would otherwise not have happened. The participants can also ask questions of each other, where something is said that they do not understand, find surprising or even with which they disagree. It is not that this makes one view wrong or another right. Rather, it provides the researcher with a wider and more diverse set of insights to which they would otherwise not have had access.

Activity 7.5   Evidence-based practice and research

Imagine you want to undertake some research in a nursing home with residents. You have the following three ideas for your project: how residents interact within the communal area; the changes a group of residents would like to see with regards to the social activities in the home; and an exploration of the individual, unique experiences of a new resident coming into the nursing home. Match the following three data collection methods to each of the three research ideas outlined above and briefly explain your choices:

- observation;
- research interview;
- focus group.

An outline answer is given at the end of the chapter.

As with all approaches, researchers must consider very carefully ethical issues. Focus groups are unlikely to be suitable where sensitive and personal issues are under consideration. For example, there is a risk that people might disclose information that they would, on reflection, have preferred not to share, and especially in a group situation. Methods are thus influenced not only by the questions that need to be answered but by the ethos of not doing harm.

Qualitative analysis

Just as there are many ways in which data can be captured in qualitative research, so the same is true for data analysis. A widely used approach is thematic analysis (Holloway and Galvin, 2017). That involves the researcher reading the transcripts and identifying emerging themes. It is not just those themes that are of interest but also occasions where insights provided by one or more participants do not sit neatly within those themes.

This provides an example of the flexibility of qualitative research. Unlike quantitative approaches, the research does not start with hypotheses to be tested. At most the researchers might have developed a set of themes they believe will be evident. However, the interviews provide opportunity for participants, in relating their perceptions and experiences, to challenge what would otherwise be taken for granted. The approach gives much greater control to participants.

In short: qualitative methods provide a means by which in-depth insights can be achieved that help understand individual experiences and understandings of social processes. They are more flexible than quantitative methods and give greater opportunity to participants to influence directions taken.

Case study: Interprofessional research

Think back to Bernadette and Abigail from Chapter 1. They are now in the final year of their studies when an exciting opportunity presents itself. They are asked to take part in a study that is designed to explore the impact of interprofessional education on communication and care standards in healthcare teams. This study used focus groups, a key social science research method that allows participants to share their experiences and perceptions in a group setting.

Bernadette and Abigail participated in several focus group discussions with a variety of healthcare professionals, including physiotherapists, podiatrists, medical students and social workers, as part of this research project. These discussions focused on the participants' interprofessional education experiences and how it affected their professional practice. Bernadette and Abigail gained first-hand knowledge of other healthcare professionals' experiences by participating in these focus groups. They heard how interprofessional education helped to break down silos, foster mutual respect and develop a shared language among professions, ultimately improving communication and patient care. They also heard about challenges, such as professionals feeling undervalued, fears of professional identity dilution, and scheduling difficulties for joint training sessions.

Bernadette and Abigail found this process of active participation in focus groups beneficial. They discovered the significance of listening to, comprehending and appreciating the perspectives of various healthcare professionals. They also recognised the complexities that underpin interprofessional collaboration, as well as the critical role that education plays in facilitating it. The findings of the focus groups shed light on the practicalities of interprofessional education and its direct implications for care standards and communication.

Activity 7.6   Critical thinking

Consider two ways that taking part in research as a participant could be beneficial to your professional development.

An outline answer is given at the end of this chapter.

Where can information relating to social science research methods be found?

There are lots of opportunities for you to better understand research that underpins the social sciences.

There are a multitude of books that provide discussion about research methods in the social sciences including some that provide accessible introductions. You are pointed to some of these in the Further Reading section at the end of this chapter. Many of these, and others, will very likely be found in your university library. It is worth looking at a few different books. Some will suit you more than others depending on your learning style. They will also give greater emphasis to particular types of research. Dip into them and ask questions of them. Don't worry if you do not understand the ideas initially. Developing your understanding is a layering process and will come over time.

A good way to develop your understanding of methods is to read a cross-section of papers in social science journals. Research papers almost always follow a similar format:

- Background: this sets out why the topic is important and the specific question or questions that the researchers set out to answer.
- Methods: this is key to understanding how the researchers set out to answer their question or questions. There should be a logical flow implicit or explicit that makes clear how the methods will provide convincing answers.
- Findings: here the researchers set out what was found.
- Discussion: the researchers explain what they see as the implications of their findings in relation to the questions initially set out. They will often acknowledge the limitations inevitable in any study and make suggestions for future research.

Journals have their own specific requirements, but this format is broadly followed in most papers. So, finding information on how the research was done is reasonably straightforward. Reading the methods in relation to other sections can help you develop your understanding of both the findings and how they were arrived at.

Like the textbooks, dip into these research papers. Don't feel that you must read them from beginning to end. Ask questions of them: what did the research set out to do? Why did the researchers think it to be important? How did they go about answering their questions?

There are a very wide range of peer-reviewed journals that report research in the social sciences. Some of these are specifically for studies that have considered health-related questions, such as *Social Science and Medicine* or the *Journal of Epidemiology and Community Health*. Others are specific to a particular branch of the social sciences, such as *Sociology of Health and Illness*. Many of the research papers reported in nursing journals, for example the *International Journal of Nursing Studies* used methods drawn from the social sciences.

Discussing research with people who do social science research can help make the topic more accessible. Take advantage of your time in university. Many of the lecturers who support your learning will have training in the social sciences. You might talk with your academic support team about research they have done or are doing and the extent to which social science methods have been used.

Keep in mind that the social sciences are themselves very broad in scope, from small ethnographic studies with a handful of interviews, up to observational studies with data relating to many thousands of people. Social scientists specialise and develop expertise in a particular discipline. While it is very possible to understand broadly different approaches, in-depth expertise is usually confined to one method. So, explore widely: speak with a range of people; read different journals. Don't be discouraged if you find it difficult. Over time and with perseverance it will come together.

Chapter summary

Understanding the evidence that lies behind the claims of the social sciences will benefit you and your practice. Even if you are not a researcher, having a knowledge of how findings were arrived at will enhance your ability to use them. It will enrich your knowledge through a more critical view on claims. You will be better placed to weigh up claims and better placed to reason. Social aspects of lives are often hidden from view and not obvious. Encouraging practice that is sensitive to the context of people's lives and long-term consequences can only be done by referring to evidence. You might be very reasonably challenged on claims you make. Understanding the research that lies behind them better places you to explain your thinking and support your contentions.

This chapter, indeed this whole book, is only a starting point. Read widely even if only dipping in. Your interest will be piqued such that you're likely to return to those papers with a questioning and critical gaze. Pick up those ideas and tell your fellow students about what you have learned. Relish those that challenge you and return to what you have read to deepen your own understanding. Over time, your knowledge of the social sciences and their application to your practice will deepen, to the benefit of your life and those of your patients.

Activities: Brief outline answers

Activity 7.1   Leadership and management

Before implementing changes, it is important to engage with research evidence related to people's experiences of admission to an acute mental health unit. This will enable you to take an evidence-based approach to care, which ensures interventions are grounded in recent, high-quality evidence, promoting effective and safe care. Furthermore, reviewing existing research can provide a comprehensive understanding of the challenges, fears and needs that people face during the admissions process, allowing for the development of strategies to specifically address these issues. By better understanding these experiences, you can increase your chances of developing interventions that are responsive to patients' needs and improve overall care quality.

Patients will all have different experiences of admission. These will be influenced by the social, geographic and economic factors listed. You might think of others. Taking these into account will assist you in thinking through steps that might be taken to support people through that period. The ways in which social background influences engagement with health services are complex, but there are key aspects that may enable different means of support to be put into place. People may be anxious about their employment situation, which would have implications for income for themselves and possibly other family members. They may be concerned about their housing status and how they will pay rent. These may be factors in why the person has required admission as well as their ongoing wellbeing while in your clinical area.

Geographical factors may also have implications for experience. For example, it may be that visiting may be more difficult for some patients' relatives given they live in a remote and rural area, especially if they are dependent on public transport. There may be issues specific to the locality in which people live that has impinged on their mental wellbeing. Perhaps they have recently relocated and have fewer support networks than previously. Thinking geographically may thus open new angles that better help you understand your patient, their situation and their concerns.

These are only examples. They are intended to act as a springboard for your thinking as to implications of social and geographic factors on your patients, people, their health and their experience of being admitted to hospital.

Activity 7.2   Evidence-based practice and research

The following provides some explanations you might use in your conversations with Jo:

1.   Trust and application of social science research in nursing:

Social science research provides valuable insights into patients' broader life contexts, which may have an impact on their health. It is critical in providing comprehensive care that extends beyond the treatment of a medical condition. It assists us in considering our patients' lifestyles, socio-economic status and other factors that may influence their health outcomes. In terms of credibility, while this type of research may not be as concrete or direct as some medical studies, it is still founded on systematic and rigorous methods. As a result, it can provide trustworthy information that can be used to improve the care we provide.

2.   Influence of sociocultural considerations on patient care:

Understanding our patients' lives outside of the hospital is critical for providing quality care. A patient living in a high-stress environment, for example, may struggle to manage a chronic disease such as diabetes or hypertension. By recognising this, we can provide more targeted stress management education, refer them to relevant social services or adjust their care plan to better suit their circumstances. Understanding these sociocultural factors allows us to not only provide better individualised care but also to advocate for our patients at a system level.

You might suggest to Jo that she reads a paper drawn from the social sciences as a basis for your discussions. The paper you use might be one you choose, or you could suggest to her that she looks through some of the journals to which she has access through her university and finds one of interest to her. You can then discuss the paper and learn together (teaching and mentoring is one of the best ways to support your own learning).

Activity 7.3   Evidence-based practice and research

There is no one answer to the question as to implications of the research findings for practice. It pays to take time to think through what you have learned and how it might impinge on the care you provide. One aspect of the 'housing first' research is that it demonstrates the links between mental health and homelessness. It also indicates that engaging with health services is challenging for people who do not have a secure tenure. One conclusion that might be drawn is that the study underlines the need to liaise closely with support services that can help people who do not have a secure tenure.

A key question when reading research is what is referred to as its 'generalisability'. To what extent can findings from a study be applied more widely. There is often no straightforward answer. Different social contexts can mean that findings are more or less applicable. Just because a study was not done in the same country or was from some time ago does not mean it cannot be drawn on. However, there are likely to be aspects in common, so should not necessarily just be dismissed. There are aspects of humanity we all share. You might look to see if other studies have been done that are more directly relevant. If not, then the study might constitute the best evidence you have.

In short, think carefully about the findings of research. Consider carefully if the study is applicable to your work. Avoid dismissing it just because it is not directly relevant.

Activity 7.4   Evidence-based practice and research

This study raises questions for nurses working in cancer care as to how they can best support people living in situations of deprivation. The reasons why survival after a cancer diagnosis is influenced by deprivation are not straightforward and embedded in wider societal processes. There may be implications for the care that you provide, however.

The study suggests that taking a social history of patients would be a good starting point. There may be factors that influence ability to engage with services that if recognised might be addressed. It is an example of the inverse care law you will have met when reading Chapter 6. A social history might be a useful means of opening conversations. There are practical issues to consider: money worries, employment and housing. Getting to appointments might be more difficult both financially and in having to take time off from work.

Ensuring patients understand what is happening and what their treatment involves is important. People living in situations of deprivation may have less confidence to speak up and ask questions. Being mindful of this can encourage you to give patients the time and space to ask questions, and to advocate for them when they are engaging with other healthcare professionals.

The research also provides a powerful means of advocating more widely, for example with your fellow students. That people die earlier predicated on their socio-economic situation is, to say the least, concerning. Findings from studies such as the one indicated here are powerful means of raising awareness and encouraging reflection and action.

Activity 7.5   Evidence-based practice and research

Here is a suggested answer matching the research project to the appropriate data collection method.

Observation: How residents interact in the communal area.

Observation is an effective data collection method for studying how residents interact in the communal area. You can gain valuable insights into their communication styles, social engagement and communal space utilisation by directly observing their behaviours, social dynamics and patterns of interaction. Observation provides a clear picture of residents' communal area experiences by providing a comprehensive understanding of their interactions.

Focus group: Changes that a group of residents would like to see in terms of social activities at the home.

A focus group would be an appropriate data collection method to investigate the changes that a group of residents would like to see in the nursing home's social activities. You can facilitate a structured discussion among a small group of residents by bringing them together. Participants can freely express their opinions, suggestions and desires for improvements in social activities. A focus group's interactive nature allows participants to build on each other's ideas, resulting in a collective perspective on the desired changes.

Research interview: Investigate the individual, one-of-a-kind experiences of a new resident entering a nursing home:

Individual research interviews would be an appropriate data collection method to explore a new resident's unique experiences upon entering the nursing home. You can delve into their personal narratives, emotions, challenges and reflections about their transition and initial experiences in the nursing home by conducting one-on-one interviews. Interviews with research participants provide a more intimate and in-depth exploration of individual perspectives, allowing for a more nuanced understanding of the new resident's journey as they settle into the home.

Activity 7.6 Critical thinking

Participating in research as a subject can benefit a healthcare professional's development in two important ways. For starters, it can broaden one's understanding of the research process by providing first-hand knowledge of ethical considerations, data collection methods and the impact of research on policy and practice. This greater comprehension can lead to a greater appreciation for the significance of research rigour, data quality and ethical research practices. Second, being a participant can improve empathy and patient-centred care significantly. It enables healthcare professionals to put themselves in the shoes of patients, understanding their experiences, anxieties and perspectives when they become research subjects. This can help the professional approach their patients with more empathy, thereby improving patient-centred care in their practice.

Further reading

Ellis, P (2022) *Understanding research for nursing students.* 5th ed. London: Sage.

This is an essential guide into research methods and terminology. It emphasises the importance of research to nursing and boosts student confidence in applying research principles to their nursing practices. The guide simplifies research terminology for beginners. Nursing students can identify high-quality research by using relatable examples and case studies, helping them to understand and evaluate current research.

Greenhalgh, T (2019) *How to read a paper: the basics of evidence-based medicine and healthcare.* 6th ed. Hoboken, NJ: Wiley Blackwell.

This is a comprehensive guide on evidence-based medicine. It guides readers with the evaluation of health literature and applying its results in practical settings. The book addresses misconceptions about evidence-based healthcare, discusses new topics like study bias and big data, and serves as a useful resource for healthcare students, practitioners and anyone looking to understand evidence-based healthcare.

Stewart, A (2016) *Basic statistics and epidemiology: a practical guide.* 4th ed. CRC Press.

This guide provides a reasonably accessible introduction to the methods used in epidemiology, including social epidemiology. You might dip into it or refer to it when reading papers that use statistics. It provides useful insights into different study designs, as well as to key statistical terms you will come across in most quantitative papers.

Dancey, CP, Reidy, J and Rowe, R (2014) *Statistics for the health sciences: A non-mathematical introduction.* London: Sage.

This book provides another reasonably accessible starting point for developing your knowledge of statistics. This book can provide you with a great basis for understanding the literature where quantitative methods have been used.

Renjith V, Yesodharan R, Noronha JA, Ladd E and George A (2021) Qualitative methods in health care research. *International Journal of Preventive Medicine*, 12(1): 20.

This article discusses qualitative research methods such as narrative research, phenomenological research, grounded theory research, ethnographic research, historical research and case study research. It is a good starting point if you are interested in qualitative research methods.

Hughes, M and Duffy, C (2018) Public involvement in health and social sciences research: A concept analysis. *Health Expect*, 21: 1183–1190.

This concept analysis is pertinent to nursing research, explores and clarifies the nature and meaning of public involvement in health and social sciences research.

Bowling, A (2023) *Research methods in health: investigating health and health services.* Maidenhead: Open University Press.

For a deeper exploration of research in the field of health, this is an accessible guide to multi-disciplinary research methods used within health and health services. It covers topics such as epidemiology, health services evaluation, health economics, and qualitative and quantitative research. You may benefit from the book's comprehensive coverage of research processes.

Useful websites

National Institute for Health and Care Research (NIHR): **www.nihr.ac.uk/**

The NIHR funds, enables and delivers world-leading health and social care research, providing resources and information on various research projects.

Centre for Behavioural Research Methods: **www.ntu.ac.uk/research/groups-and-centres/centres/centre-for-behavioural-research-methods**

The theory and practice of social science research methods are nurtured, developed and shared through this interdisciplinary hub at Nottingham Trent University.

RCN Research Society: **www.rcn.org.uk/Get-Involved/Forums/Research-Society**

The Society provides research guidance to help the Royal College of Nursing shape evidence-based practices and meet members' needs. It is also involved in establishing a network for sharing experiences and fostering learning opportunities.

The Economic and Social Research Council (ESRC): **www.ukri.org/councils/esrc/**

The ESRC are the major funders of the social sciences in the United Kingdom. The research they fund includes health-focused work as well as studies with broader societal interests (as you will have learned in this book, those wider determinants are often key health determinants).

Conclusion

This book has examined the important role that social sciences play in shaping the nursing profession and its practices. We have investigated the origins of social sciences, demonstrating how they provide a foundation for exploring the complex interplay between individuals, communities and the healthcare system. You hopefully feel better prepared for the multifaceted aspects of nursing practice. We have shown how an understanding of the social sciences helps recognise why holistic care and the biopsychosocial approach in nursing are important. You will become a more effective nurse by considering the biological, psychological and social factors that influence health and wellbeing.

The recognition of inequalities and discrimination that persist within healthcare settings has been a major theme in this book. We hope this has raised your awareness about the critical need for culturally competent care by investigating the factors that contribute to these disparities, such as race, gender, socio-economic status and cultural backgrounds. Nursing professionals with this knowledge can advocate for change, aiming to create a more equitable and just healthcare system for all. This may include approaches towards activism and politics in the nursing profession. Nurses hold a unique position within the healthcare system, allowing them to be powerful change agents. During your career, you can help shape public discourse and contribute to the implementation of health policies that promote social justice and improved population health outcomes by engaging in advocacy, policy development and community activism.

Another central theme of this book has been population health, emphasising the importance of nursing professionals understanding the social determinants of health and the broader factors that influence wellbeing and health outcomes. You have learned how to contribute to the development of approaches that address the root causes of health disparities by drawing on knowledge from the social sciences. The final stages of the book have shown you the importance of social science research in nursing, demonstrating how it can inform evidence-based practice, drive improvements in patient care, and contribute to the nursing profession's ongoing development. Nurses can broaden their knowledge and contribute to the evidence base that underpins nursing practice by engaging in and conducting social science research.

To summarise, the purpose of this book was to demonstrate the importance of social sciences in nursing education and practice. We hope it has shown how nursing's complex and multidimensional nature can be grasped through engagement with these disciplines. As we come to the end of this journey, we hope that anyone reading this book now has a better understanding of the social sciences and their vital contributions to the nursing profession. We encourage readers to keep exploring these disciplines and embrace the knowledge and insights they provide to enhance their practice and advocate for change. Together we can make a difference in creating a more equitable and compassionate healthcare future. Beyond all else, we hope you can see the value of incorporating curiosity and critical thinking into your nursing practice.

References

Adriaansen, M, Van Achterberg, T and Borm, G (2008). The usefulness of the staff-patient interaction response scale for palliative care nursing for measuring the empathetic capacity of nursing students. *Journal of Professional Nursing*, 24(5): 315–323. https://doi.org/10.1016/j.profnurs.2007.10.003

Advance HE (2020) We stand united against racism. [Online] Available: www.advance-he.ac.uk/we-stand-united-against-racism [Accessed: 23 April 2022]

Agnew, T (2016) An extraordinary life. *Nursing Standard*, 31(6): 22–25. https://doi.org/10.7748/ns.31.6.22.s24

Alasuutari, P, Bickman, L and Brannen, J (2008). *The SAGE handbook of social research methods*. SAGE Publications Ltd. https://doi.org/10.4135/9781446212165

Allen, D (2021) Hairstyles, hostility and the prejudice Black nurses can face about their locs. *Nursing Standard*, 36(7): 35–37. https://doi.org/10.7748/ns.36.7.35.s17

All-Party Parliamentary Group (2021) Sickle cell and thalassaemia. [Online] Available: https://publications.parliament.uk/pa/cm/cmallparty/211117/sickle-cell-and-thalassaemia.htm [Accessed: 22 June 2023]

Almirall, J, Serra-Prat, M, Bolíbar, I and Balasso, V (2017). Risk factors for community-acquired pneumonia in adults: a systematic review of observational studies. *Respiration*, 94(3): 299–311.

American Sociological Association (2019) What is sociology? [Online] Available: www.asanet.org/about/what-sociology [Accessed: 22 February 2022]

Andermann, A (2018). Screening for social determinants of health in clinical care: moving from the margins to the mainstream. *Public Health Reviews*, 39: 1–17.

Arabi, A, Rafi, F, Cheraghi, MA and Ghiyasvandian, S (2014) Nurses' policy influence: a concept analysis. *Iranian Journal of Nursing and Midwifery Research*, 13(3): 315–322.

Aranda, K and Law, K (2007). Tales of sociology and the nursing curriculum: revisiting the debates. *Nurse Education Today*, 27(6): 561–567. https://doi.org/10.1016/j.nedt.2006.08.017

Archibong, U, Kline, R, Eshareturi, C and McIntosh, B (2019). Disrupting disproportionality proceedings: the recommendations. *British Journal of Health Care Management*, 25(6): 1–6. https://doi.org/10.12968/bjhc.2018.0063

Artiga, S and Hinton, E (2018) Beyond health care: the role of social determinants in promoting health and health equity. *Issue Brief*. www.kff.org/racial-equity-and-health-policy/

issue-brief/beyond-health-care-the-role-of-social-determinants-in-promoting-health-and-health-equity/ [Accessed: 21 September 2022]

Atherton, IM and Kyle, RG (2014) Learn to see patients in their world. *Nursing Standard*, 28(50): 22–24.

Aubry, T, Tsemberis, S, Adair, CE, Veldhuizen, S, Streiner, D, Latimer, E, Sareen, J, Patterson, M, McGarvey, K, Kopp, B and Hume, C (2015) One-year outcomes of a randomized controlled trial of housing first with ACT in five Canadian cities. *Psychiatric Services*, 66(5): 463–469.

Ayala, RA (2020). *Towards a sociology of nursing*. Singapore: Palgrave MacMillan.

Bambra, C, Riordan, R, Ford, J, and Matthews, F (2020). The COVID-19 pandemic and health inequalities. *Journal of Epidemiology and Community Health*, 74(11): 964–968. https://doi.org/10.1136/jech-2020-214401

Barr, J and Dowding, L (2022) *Leadership in health care*. 5th ed. London: Sage.

Baumgartner, LM and Johnson-Bailey, J (2008) Fostering awareness of diversity and multiculturalism in adult and higher education. *New Directions for Adult and Continuing Education*, 120, 45–53.

Blackmore, C (2010) *Social learning systems and communities of practice*. London: Springer.

Blaxter, M (1997) Whose fault is it? People's own conceptions of the reasons for health inequalities. *Social Science and Medicine*, 44(6): 747–756.

Boswell, C, Cannon, SB and Miller, J (2013). Students' perceptions of holistic nursing care. *Nursing Education Perspectives*, 34(5): 329–333.

Bowling, A (2023) *Research methods in health: investigating health and health services*. 5th ed. Maidenhead: Open University Press.

Briggs, EC, Amaya-Jackson, L, Putnam, KT and Putnam, FW (2021) All adverse childhood experiences are not equal: the contribution of synergy to adverse childhood experience scores. *American Psychologist*, 76(2): 243–252.

Brinkmann, S and Kvale, S (2015) *Interviews: learning the craft of qualitative research interviewing*. 3rd ed. London: Sage Publications.

British Geriatrics Society (2019) www.bgs.org.uk/resources/resource-series/comprehensive-geriatric-assessment-toolkit-for-primary-care-practitioners [Accessed: 5 June 2022]

The British Psychological Association (2019) Adverse childhood experiences [Online] Available: https://cms.bps.org.uk/sites/default/files/2022-06/Briefing%20Paper%20-%20Adverse%20Childhood%20Experiences_0.pdf [Accessed: 10 September 2023]

British Sociological Association (2022) What do sociologists do? [Online] Available: www.britsoc.co.uk/what-is-sociology/what-do-sociologists-do/ [Accessed: 22 February 2022]

Brodsky, AE and Marx, CM (2001) Layers of identity: multiple psychological senses of community within a community setting. *Journal of Community Psychology*, 29(2): 161–178.

Brown, MJ, Kaur, A, James, T, Avalos, C, Addo, PNO, Crouch, E and Hill, NL (2022) Adverse childhood experiences and subjective cognitive decline in the US. *Journal of Applied Gerontology*, 41(4): 1090–1100.

Buck-McFadyen, E and MacDonnell, J (2017) Contested practice: political activism in nursing and implications for nursing education. *International Journal of Nursing Education Scholarship*, 14(1): 743–761.

Buckner, S, Darlington, N, Woodward, M, Buswell, M, Mathie, E, Arthur, A, Lafortune, L, Killett, A, Mayrhofer, A, Thurman, J and Goodman, C (2019) Dementia friendly communities in England: a scoping study. *International Journal of Geriatric Psychiatry*, 34(8): 1235–1243.

Campbell, K (2022) Towards an anti-racist curriculum. [Online] Available: https://gcuacaddevelopment.wordpress.com/2022/01/10/towards-an-anti-racist-curriculum/ [Accessed: 10 May 2022]

Chapman, H (2017) Nursing theories 1: person-centred care. *Nursing Times*, 113(10): 59.

Chase, E and Walker, R (2013) The co-construction of shame in the context of poverty: beyond a threat to the social bond. *Sociology*, 47(4): 739–754.

Christianson, KL (2020) Emotional intelligence and critical thinking in nursing students: integrative review of literature. *Nurse Educator*, 45(6): E62–E65.

Cohen N and Galea S (2011) *Population mental health*. Abingdon: Routledge

Conoley, C, Pontrelli, ME, Oromendia, MF, Carmen Bello, BD and Nagata, CM (2015) Positive empathy: a therapeutic skill inspired by positive psychology: Positive Empathy. *Journal of Clinical Psychology*, 71(6): 575–583. https://doi.org/10.1002/jclp.22175

Cowling, W (2020) Systemic racism and holistic nursing: a start. *Journal of Holistic Nursing*, 38(3): 260–262.

Cox, G, Sobrany, S, Jenkins, E, Musipa, C and Darbyshire, P (2021) Time for nursing to eradicate hair discrimination. *Journal of Clinical Nursing*, 30(9–10): e45–e47.

Creswell, JW and Poth, CN (2018) *Qualitative inquiry and research design: choosing among five approaches*. 4th ed. London: Sage Publications.

Crow, G (2014) The sociology of community. In: Holmwood, J and Scott, J (eds) *The Palgrave handbook of sociology in Britain*. London: Palgrave Macmillan. https://doi.org/10.1057/9781137318862_17

Dahlgren and Whitehead (1993), cited in Dahlgren, G and Whitehead, M, 2021. The Dahlgren-Whitehead model of health determinants: 30 years on and still chasing rainbows. *Public Health*, 199: 20–24.

Dana, R and Upton, D (2013) *Psychology for nurses*. Harlow: Pearson Education Limited.

Davies, R (2012) Ivan Illich on medical nemesis. *Nurse Education Today*, 32(1): 5–6.

Devereux, E (2022) Nurse activist calls on colleagues to 'stand up' to climate crisis. [Online] Available: www.nursingtimes.net/news/sustainability-and-environment/nurse-activist-calls-on-colleagues-to-stand-up-to-climate-crisis-08-12-2022/ [Accessed: 8 March 2023]

Digital Poverty Alliance (2022) Directory for support [Online] Available: https://digitalpovertyalliance.org/dpa-directory-for-support/ [Accessed: 1 February 2022]

Disch and Kingston (2021) Using activism to get nurses on boards. *Nursing Administration Quarterly*, 45(3): 208–218. doi: 10.1097/NAQ.0000000000000474.

Doherty, C, Dooley, K and Woods, A (2013) Teaching sociology within teacher education: revisiting, realigning and re-embedding. *Journal of Sociology*, 49(4): 515–530.

Dossey, BM and Dossey, L (1998) Body-mind-spirit: attending to holistic care. *The American Journal of Nursing*, 98(8): 35–38. https://doi.org/10.2307/3471907. [Accessed 1 September 2022]

Dubet, F (2021) The return of society. *European Journal of Social Theory*, 24(1): 3–21.

Economic and Social Research Council (2023) Consent. [Online] Available: www.ukri.org/councils/esrc/guidance-for-applicants/research-ethics-guidance/consent/ [Accessed 12 June 2023]

Edgley, A, Timmons, S and Crosbie, B (2009) Desperately seeking sociology: nursing student perceptions of sociology on nursing courses. *Nurse Education Today*, 29(1): 16–23. https://doi.org/10.1016/j.nedt.2008.06.001

Eijkelboom, Brouwers, M, Frenkel, J, van Gurp, P, Jaarsma, D, de Jonge, R, Koksma, J, Mulder, D, Schaafsma, E, Sehlbach, C, Warmenhoven, F, Willemen, A and de la Croix, A (2023) Twelve tips for patient involvement in health professions education. *Patient Education and Counseling*, 106: 92–97. https://doi.org/10.1016/j.pec.2022.09.016

Ellis, P (2022) *Understanding research for nursing students.* 5th ed. London: Sage

Engel, GL (1977) The need of a new medical model: a challenge for bioscience. *Science*, 196: 129–136

Equal Opportunities Commission, (2022) What is discrimination? [Online] www.eoc.org.uk/what-is-discrimination/ [Accessed: 1 April 2023]

Equality Act (2010) [Online] Available: www.legislation.gov.uk/ukpga/2010/15/contents [Accessed: 21 April 2020]

Equality and Human Rights Commission (2019) Tackling racial harassment: universities challenged. [Online] Available: www.equalityhumanrights.com/sites/default/files/tackling-racial-harassment-universities-challenged.pdf [Accessed: 1 May 2022]

Essex, R and Weldon, SM (2022) The justification for strike action in healthcare: a systematic critical interpretive synthesis. *Nursing ethics*, 29(5): 1152–1173. https://doi.org/10.1177/09697330211022411

Etowa, J (2016) Diversity, racism and Eurocentric-normative practice in healthcare. *International Journal of Health Sciences and Research*, 6 (January): 278–289.

Fadol, A, Estrella, J, Shelton, V, Zaghian, M, Vanbenschop, D, Counts, V, Mendoza, TR, Rubio, D and Johnston, PA (2019) A quality improvement approach to reducing hospital readmissions in patients with cancer and heart failure. *Cardio-oncology (London)*, 5, 5. https://doi.org/10.1186/s40959-019-0041-x

FEANTSA (2017) ETHOS: A European typology of homelessness and housing exclusion. European Federation of National Organisations Working with the Homeless. www.feantsa.org/en/toolkit/2005/04/01/ethos-typology-on-homelessness-and-housing-exclusion [Accessed 2 August 2023]

Finn, V Stephenson, J and Astin, F (2018) Patient preferences for involvement in health service development. *British Journal of Nursing*, 27(17): 1004–1010. https://doi.org/10.12968/bjon.2018.27.17.1004

FitzGerald, C and Hurst, S (2017) Implicit bias in healthcare professionals: a systematic review. *BMC Medical Ethics*, 18(1): 19. https://doi.org/10.1186/s12910-017-0179-8

Florell, MC (2021) Concept analysis of nursing activism. *Nursing Forum*, 56(1): 134–140. https://doi.org/10.1111/nuf.12502

Forrest, S (2016) A Core Curriculum for Sociology in UK undergraduate medical education. A report from the Behavioural and Social Sciences Teaching in Medicine (BeSST) Sociology Steering Group. Cardiff: Cardiff University.

Fowler, M (2017) 'Unladylike commotion': early feminism and nursing's role in gender/trans dialogue. *Nurs Inq*, 24: e12179. https://doi.org/10.1111/nin.12179

Friedli, L (2013) What we've tried, hasn't worked: The politics of assets based public health 1. *Critical Public Health*, 23(2): 131–145. https://doi.org/10.1080/09581596.2012.748882

Frisch, NC and Rabinowitsch, D (2019) What's in a definition? holistic nursing, integrative health care, and integrative nursing: report of an integrated literature review. *Journal of Holistic Nursing*, 37(3): 260–272.

Giddens, A and Sutton, PW (2021) *Sociology*. 9th ed. Cambridge: Polity Press.

Gilliver, C (2018) Trauma-informed care in response to adverse childhood experiences. *Nursing Times*, 114(7): 46–49.

Göl, İ and Erkin, Ö (2019) Association between cultural intelligence and cultural sensitivity in nursing students: a cross-sectional descriptive study. *Collegian*, 26(4): 485–491. https://doi.org/10.1016/j.colegn.2018.12.007

Goodman, B (2013) Erving Goffman and the total institution. *Nurse Education Today*, 33(2): 81–82. https://doi.org/10.1016/j.nedt.2012.09.012

Goodman, B and Grant, A (2017) The case of the Trump regime: the need for resistance in international nurse education. *Nurse Education Today*, 52: 53–56.

Gray, AJ (2011) Worldviews. *International Psychology*, 8(3): 58–60. Available: www.ncbi.nlm.nih.gov/pmc/articles/PMC6735033/

Grealish, L and Ranse, K (2009) An exploratory study of first year nursing students' learning in the clinical workplace. *Contemporary Nurse*, 33(1): 80–92.

Green, C (2021) Teaching the history of psychology. *Canadian Psychology/Psychologie Canadienne*, 62(4): 400–408.

Greenhalgh, T (2019) *How to read a paper: the basics of evidence-based medicine and healthcare.* 6th ed. Hoboken, NJ: Wiley Blackwell.

Gregory, A, Walker, M and Anonson, J (2022). Social media and nursing activism: a literature review. *Canadian Journal of Nursing Informatics*, 17(2): 1–13. https://cjni.net/journal/?p=10088

Grønning, K, Karlsholm, G and André, B (2022) Undergraduate nursing students' experiences of conducting clinical research projects in their bachelor theses – a qualitative study. *SAGE Open Nursing*, 8: 23779608221094537. https://doi.org/10.1177/23779608221094537

Gross, R (2020) *Psychology: the science of mind and behaviour.* 8th ed. London: Hodder Education.

Haralambos, M, Holborn, M, Chapman, S and Moore, S (2013) *Sociology: themes and perspectives.* 8th ed. London: Collins.

Harris, J and Nimmo, S (2013) *Placement learning in community nursing.* Edinburgh: Elsevier.

The Health Foundation (2022) Addressing the leading risk factors for ill health: A review of government policies tackling smoking, poor diet, physical inactivity and harmful alcohol use in England [Online] Available: www.health.org.uk/publications/reports/addressing-the-leading-risk-factors-for-ill-health [Accessed: 19 June 2023]

Heaslip, V, Thompson, R, Tauringana, M, Holland, S and Glendening, N (2022) Health inequity in the UK: exploring health inequality and inequity. *Practice Nursing*, 33(2): 72–76.

Helming, MAB, Shields, DA, Avino, KM and Rosa, WE (2020) *Dossey and Keegan's holistic nursing: a handbook for practice.* 8th ed. Redhill: Jones and Bartlett Learning.

Henry, R, Hartley, B, Simpson, M and Doyle, N (2014) The development and evaluation of a holistic needs assessment and care planning learning package targeted at cancer nurses in the UK. *Ecancermedicalscience*, 8(1): 1–6. https://doi.org/10.3332/ecancer.2014.416

Holloway, I and Galvin, K (2017) *Qualitative research in nursing and healthcare.* 4th ed. Chichester: John Wiley.

Hughes, M and Duffy, C (2018) Public involvement in health and social sciences research: a concept analysis. *Health Expect*, 21(6): 1183–1190. https://doi.org/10.1111/hex.12825

Ingleby, FC, Woods, LM, Atherton, IM, Baker, M, Elliss-Brookes, L and Belot, A (2022) An investigation of cancer survival inequalities associated with individual-level socio-economic status, area-level deprivation, and contextual effects, in a cancer patient cohort in England and Wales. *BMC Public Health*, 22(1): 90. https://doi.org/10.1186/s12889-022-12525-1

Institute of Health Equity (2013) Working for health equity: the role of health care professionals. Institute of Health Equity, London. [Online] Available: www.instituteofhealthequity.org/resources-reports/working-for-health-equity-the-role-of-health-professionals/working-for-health-equity-the-role-of-health-professionals-full-report.pdf [Accessed: 4 April 2023]

Institute of Health Equity (2021) equity-covid-19-and-the-social-determinants-of-health-sdh.pdf (instituteofhealthequity.org) COVID-19 2021 (October).

Jacobsen, KH (2021) *Introduction to health research methods: a practical guide.* Burlington: Jones & Bartlett Learning.

Jasemi, M, Valizadeh, L, Zamanzadeh, V and Keogh, B (2017) A concept analysis of holistic care by hybrid model. *Indian Journal of Palliative Care*, 23(1): 71–78.

Jazi, ZH, Gheybi, K, Zare, Z and Shahsavari, H (2022) Nursing students' experiences of educational discrimination: a qualitative study. *BMC Nursing*, 21(1): 1–7.

Kamper, A, Chiarotto, A, Smeets, RJE, Ostelo, RWJ, Guzman, J and van Tulder, M (2015) Multidisciplinary biopsychosocial rehabilitation for chronic low back pain: Cochrane systematic review and meta-analysis. *BMJ*, 350, h444–h444. https://doi.org/10.1136/bmj.h444

Kindig, D and Stoddart, G (2003) What is population health? *American Journal of Public Health*, 93(3): 380–383.

King's Fund (2022a) What is happening to life expectancy in England? The King's Fund (kingsfund.org.uk).

King's Fund (2022b) What is a population health approach? www.kingsfund.org.uk/publications/population-health-approach [Accessed: 14 April 2023]

King's Fund (2022c) What are health inequalities. [Online] Available: www.kingsfund.org.uk/publications/what-are-health-inequalities [Accessed: 5 May 2023]

Kinney, P (2017) Walking interviews. Social Science Update SRU 67. University of Surrey: SRU67.pdf (surrey.ac.uk)

Kirkebøen, G (2019) Descartes on emotions, reason, and the adaptive unconscious: the pioneer behind the caricature. *History of Psychology*, 22(1): 17–39.

Koch, TF, Leal, VJ and Ayala, RA (2016) Let's talk about society: a critical discourse analysis of sociology courses in pre-registration nursing. *Nurse Education Today*, 36: 139–144. https://doi.org/10.1016/j.nedt.2015.09.003

Kuehnert, P, Fawcett, J, DePriest, K, Chinn, P, Cousin, L, Ervin, N, Flanagan, J, Fry-Bowers, E, Killion, C, Maliski, S and Maughan, ED (2022) Defining the social determinants of health for nursing action to achieve health equity: a consensus paper from the American Academy of Nursing. *Nursing Outlook*, 70(1): 10–27.

Lave, J and Wenger, E (1991) *Situated learning: legitimate peripheral participation.* Cambridge: Cambridge University Press.

Lee, A and Padilla, C (2022) Causes of health inequities. *Current Opinion in Anesthesiology*, 35(3): 278–284.

Lin, SY (2017) Dementia-friendly communities' and being dementia friendly in healthcare settings. *Current Opinion in Psychiatry*, 30(2): 145–150.

Linsley, P and Roll, C (2023) *Health promotion for nursing students.* London: Sage.

Lipscomb, M (ed.) (2017) *Social theory and nursing.* London: Taylor and Francis.

Lyndon, H, Latour, JM, Marsden, J, Campbell, S, Stevens, K and Kent, B (2019) The holistic assessment and care planning in partnership intervention study (HAPPI): A protocol for a feasibility, cluster randomised controlled trial. *Journal of Advanced Nursing*, 75(11): 3078–3087. https://doi.org/10.1111/jan.14106

Mackenbach, JP, Stirbu, I, Roskam, AJR, Schaap, MM, Menvielle, G, Leinsalu, M and Kunst, AE (2008) Socioeconomic inequalities in health in 22 European countries. *New England Journal of Medicine*, 358(23): 2468–2481.

Major, D (2019) Developing effective nurse leadership skills. *Nursing Standard*. https://doi.org/10.7748/ns.2019.e11247

Marmot, M (2016) *The health gap: improving health in an unequal world.* London: Bloomsbury.

Marmot, M (2018) An inverse care law for our time. *BMJ*, 362.

Marshall, K and Easton, C (2018) The role of asset-based approaches in community nursing. *Primary Health Care*, 28(5): 35–38. https://doi.org/10.7748/phc.2018.e1339

Maslow, AH (1943) A theory of human motivation. *Psychological Review*, 50(4): 370–396.

Matsuoka, S (2021) Recovery-oriented nursing care based on cultural sensitivity in community psychiatric nursing. *International Journal of Mental Health Nursing*, 30(2): 563–573. https://doi.org/10.1111/inm.12822

Matthews, D (2015a) Part 1 of 5: Sociology in nursing. *Nursing Times*, 111(41): 18–20.

Matthews, D (2015b) Part 2 of 5: Social class and its influence on health. *Nursing Times*, 111(42): 20–21.

McCartney, G, Popham, F, McMaster, R and Cumbers, A (2019) Defining health and health inequalities. *Public Health*, 172: 22–30. https://doi.org/10.1016/j.puhe.2019.03.023

McCormack, B and McCance, T (2016) *Person-centred practice in nursing and health care.* 2nd ed. Chichester: Wiley Blackwell.

McGrath, C, Palmgren, PJ and Liljedahl, M (2019) Twelve tips for conducting qualitative research interviews. *Medical Teacher*, 41(9): 1002–1006. Available: https://doi.org/10.1080/0142159X.2018.1497149

McKendrick, JH (1999) Multi-method research: an introduction to its application in population geography. *Professional Geographer*, 51(1): 40–50.

McPherson, NG (2008) The role of sociology in nurse education: a call for consistency. *Nurse Education Today*, 28(6): 653–656.

Mental Health Foundation (2021) www.mentalhealth.org.uk/explore-mental-health/a-z-topics/stigma-and-discrimination [Accessed: 21 September 2022]

Ministry of Justice (2021) Ethnicity and the criminal justice system, 2020 [Online] Available: www.gov.uk/government/statistics/ethnicity-and-the-criminal-justice-system-statistics-2020/ethnicity-and-the-criminal-justice-system-2020 [Accessed: 15 May 2022]

Molesworth, M (2017) Nursing Students' First Placement: peripherality and marginality within the community of practice. *Journal of Nursing Education*, 56(1): 31–38. https://doi.org/10.3928/01484834-20161219-07

Molesworth, M and Lewitt, M (2019) Sociology in UK nurse education curricula: a review of the literature from 1919–2019. *Social Theory and Health*, 17: 427–442.

Morgan, A and Ziglio, E (2007) Revitalising the evidence base for public health: an assets model. *Promotion and Education*, Suppl 2: 17–22. https://doi.org/10.1177/10253823070140020701x

Mowforth, G, Harrison, J and Morris, M (2005) An investigation into adult nursing students' experience of the relevance and application of behavioural sciences (biology, psychology and sociology) across two different curricula. *Nurse Education Today*, 25(1): 41–48.

Mulgan, G (2019) *Social innovation: how societies find the power to change.* Bristol: Policy Press.

Murji, K, Neal, S and Solomos, J (2022) *Introduction to sociology.* London: Sage.

Nairn, S, Hardy, C, Harling, M, Parumal, L and Narayanasamy, M (2012) Diversity and ethnicity in nurse education: the perspective of nurse lecturers. *Nurse Education Today*, 32(3): 203–207. https://doi.org/10.1016/j.nedt.2011.02.012

National Institute for Clinical Excellence (2019) Evidence for strengths and asset-based outcomes. [Online] Available: https://www.nice.org.uk/about/nice-communities/social-care/quick-guides/evidence-for-strengths-and-asset-based-outcomes [Accessed: 10 September 2023]

National Institute for Clinical Excellence (2021) Chest infections – adult: scenario: community-acquired pneumonia. [Online] Available: https://cks.nice.org.uk/topics/chest-infections-adult/management/community-acquired-pneumonia/ [Accessed: 2 August 2023]

National Records of Scotland (2021) Life expectancy in Scotland, 2018–2020. [Online] Available: www.nrscotland.gov.uk/statistics-and-data/statistics/statistics-by-theme/life-expectancy/life-expectancy-in-scotland/2018-2020 [Accessed: 21 March 2023]

Newman, DM (2014) *Sociology: exploring the architecture of everyday life.* London: Sage.

NHS (2019a) The NHS long term plan [Online] Available: www.longtermplan.nhs.uk/ [Accessed: 16 June 2023]

NHS (2019b) Digital inclusion guide for health and social care. [Online] Available: https://digital.nhs.uk/binaries/content/assets/website-assets/corporate-information/inclusion-guide-documents/downloadable-digital-inclusion-guide.pdf [Accessed: 8 April 2022]

NHS (2021) Health literacy. [Online] Available: https://service-manual.nhs.uk/content/health-literacy [Accessed: 20 March 2022]

NHS Greater Glasgow and Clyde (2017) Director of public health report. [Online] Available: https://www.stor.scot.nhs.uk/bitstream/handle/11289/579737/Back+to+Basics+-+DPH+Report+2015.pdf?sequence=1 [Accessed: 19 September 2023]

NHS Health Education England (2023) Health literacy toolkit. [Online] Available: https://library.nhs.uk/wp-content/uploads/sites/4/2023/06/Health-Literacy-Toolkit.pdf [Accessed: 10 September 2023]

NHS Health Education England (2023) Psychology [Online] Available: https://learning-disability.hee.nhs.uk/careers/find-a-role-to-suit-you/psychology/ [Accessed: 10 September 2023].

NHS Race and Health Observatory (2022) [Online] Available: www.manchester.ac.uk/discover/news/services/downloadfile.php?f=rho-rapid-review-final-report-v.7.pdf&uid=1139877&hash=8c1f63a90532ae3ede061168dad317e77b0447d6 [Accessed: 22 June 2023]

Nurses' Registration Act (1919) [Online] Available: https://navigator.health.org.uk/content/nurses-registration-act-1919 [Accessed: 2 June 2018]

Nursing and Midwifery Council (2018a) Part 3: standards for pre-registration nursing programmes. [Online] Available: www.nmc.org.uk/globalassets/sitedocuments/standards-of-proficiency/standards-for-pre-registration-nursing-programmes/programme-standards-nursing.pdf [Accessed: 26 October 2018]

Nursing and Midwifery Council (2018b) *Future nurse: standards of proficiency for registered nurses.* London: Nursing and Midwifery Council.

Nursing and Midwifery Council (2018c) *The code: professional standards of practice and behaviour for nurses, midwives and nurse associates.* 2nd ed. London: NMC. [Accessed: 19 June 2023]

Nursing and Midwifery Council (2020a) Person-centred care. [Online] Available: www.nmc.org.uk/standards/code/code-in-action/person-centred-care/ [Accessed: 2 April 2022]

Nursing and Midwifery Council (2020b) Being inclusive and challenging discrimination [Online] Available: www.nmc.org.uk/standards/code/code-in-action/inclusivity/ [Accessed: 15 February 2023]

Nursing and Midwifery Council (2022a) Audience insight research. [Online] Available: www.nmc.org.uk/globalassets/sitedocuments/other-publications/audience-insight-research-2022.pdf [Accessed: 22 June 2023]

Nursing and Midwifery Council (2022b) Social media guidance. [Online] Available: www.nmc.org.uk/globalassets/sitedocuments/nmc-publications/social-media-guidance.pdf [Accessed: 22 June 2023]

Office for National Statistics (2021) National life tables – life expectancy in the UK: 2018 to 2020. National life tables life expectancy in the UK 2018 to 2020. [Online] Available: https://www.ons.gov.uk/peoplepopulationandcommunity/birthsdeathsandmarriages/lifeexpectancies/bulletins/nationallifetablesunitedkingdom/2018to2020 [Accessed: 31 March 2021]

Ojemeni, Jun, J, Porsen, C, Cerchow, L, Arneson, G, Orofo, C, Nava, A and Squires, AP (2023) A scoping review of nursing and midwifery activism in the United States. *Online Journal of Issues in Nursing,* 28(2): 1–15.

Olusoga, D (2017) *Black and British: a forgotten history.* London: Picador Books.

Percy, M and Richardson, C (2018) Introducing nursing practice to student nurses: how can we promote care compassion and empathy. *Nurse Education in Practice,* 29(March 2017): 200–205. https://doi.org/10.1016/j.nepr.2018.01.008

Pérez-Sánchez, S, Madueño, SE and Montaner, J (2021) Gender gap in the leadership of health institutions: the influence of hospital-level factors. *Health equity,* 5(1): 521–525. https://doi.org/10.1089/heq.2021.0013

Pérez-Wilson, P, Marcos-Marcos, J, Morgan, A, Eriksson, M, Lindström, B and Álvarez-Dardet, C (2020) 'A synergy model of health': an integration of salutogenesis and the health assets model. *Health Promotion International*, Advance Article, 1–1.

Price, B (2021) *Critical thinking and writing in nursing*. 5th ed. Exeter: Learning Matters.

Pujolar, G, Oliver-Anglès, A, Vargas, I and Vázquez, ML (2022) Changes in access to health services during the COVID-19 pandemic: a scoping review. International *Journal of Environmental Research and Public Health*, 19(3): 1749–80. https://doi.org/10.3390/ijerph19031749

Punch, S Harden, J Marsh, I and Keating, M (2013) *Sociology: making sense of society*. 5th ed. London: Pearson

Rafii, F, Ghezeljeh, T and Nasrollah, S (2019) Discriminative nursing care: a grounded theory study. *Journal of Family Medicine and Primary Care*, 8(7): 2289–2293.

Rahman, S and Swaffer, K (2018) Assets-based approaches and dementia-friendly communities. *Dementia: The International Journal of Social Research and Practice* 17(2): 131–137.

Refugee Council (2023) Mental health support for refugee women. [Online] Available: www.refugeecouncil.org.uk/our-work/mental-health-support-for-refugees-and-asylum-seekers/mental-health-support-for-refugee-women/ [Accessed: 22 June 2023]

Renjith V, Yesodharan R, Noronha JA, Ladd E and George A (2021) Qualitative methods in health care research. *International Journal of Preventative Medicine*, 12(20): 1–7. https://www.ijpvmjournal.net/text.asp?2021/12/1/20/310141 [Accessed 21 September 2023]

Rippon, S and Hopkins, T (2015) Head, hands and heart: asset-based approaches in health care [Online] Available: www.health.org.uk/publications/head-hands-and-heart-asset-based-approaches-in-health-care [Accessed: 8 April 2022]

Rowlands, G, Protheroe, J, Winkleym, J, Richardson, M, Seed, PT and Rudd, R (2015) A mismatch between population health literacy and the complexity of health information: an observational study. *British Journal of General Practice*, 65(635): e379–386. https://doi.org/10.3399/bjgp15X685285

Royal College of Nursing (2012) The Willis commission: quality with compassion – the future of nursing education. (Chairman Lord Willis of Knaresborough) London: Royal College of Nursing.

Royal College of Nursing (2019) Communication and empathy. www.rcn.org.uk/centenary/projects/100-top-tips/communication-and-empathy [Accessed: 14 June 2022]

Royal College of Nursing (2023) RCN campaigns. Available at: https://www.rcn.org.uk/Get-Involved/Campaign-with-us/Fair-Pay-for-Nursing [Accessed: 21 September 2023]

Ruddick, F (2010) Person-centred mental health care: myth or reality? *Mental Health Practice*, 13(9): 24–28.

Sanders, C (2019) Cartographers of disrupted belonging: Sudanese mothers drawing maps of Portsmouth (UK). *Journal of International Women's Studies*, 20(4), 5–23.

Sandsund, C, Towers, R, Thomas, K, Tigue, R, Lalji, A, Fernandes, A, Doyle, N, Jordan, J, Gage, H and Shaw, C (2020) Holistic needs assessment and care plans for women with gynaecological cancer: do they improve cancer-specific health-related quality of life? A randomised controlled trial using mixed methods. *BMJ Supportive and Palliative Care*, 10(2): 1–14. https://doi.org/10.1136/bmjspcare-2016-001207

Scambler, G (2012) Health inequalities. *Sociology of Health and Illness*, 34(1): 130–146.

Scheffer, MMJ, Lasater, K, Atherton, IM and Kyle, RG (2019) Student nurses' attitudes to social justice and poverty: an international comparison. *Nurse Education Today*, 80: 59–66. https://doi.org/10.1016/j.nedt.2019.06.007

Scottish Government (2019a) Revaluation of the family nurse partnership in Scotland. [Online] Available: www.gov.scot/publications/revaluation-family-nurse-partnership-scotland/ [Accessed: 14 June 2022]

Scottish Government (2019b) No One Left Behind (NOLB) employability funding stream. [Online] Available: www.gov.scot/publications/no-one-left-behind-funding-stream-equality-impact-assessment-summary/ [Accessed: 10 November 2019]

Scottish Government (2020) Evaluation of the Family Nurse Partnership in Scotland. [Online] Available: www.gov.scot/publications/evaluation-family-nurse-partnership-scotland-methods-paper-process-success-linkages/pages/2/ [Accessed: 14 June 2022]

Scottish Government (2021) 10-year anniversary publication for the Family Nurse Partnership. [Online] Available: www.gov.scot/publications/fnp-10-year-anniversary-publication-family-nurses-perspective/ [Accessed: 14 June 2022]

Sen, A (1998) Mortality as an indicator of economic success and failure. *The Economic Journal*, 108(446): 1–25.

Seteanu, S and Giosan, C (2021) Adverse childhood experiences in fathers and the consequences in their children. *Professional Psychology: Research and Practice*, 52(1): 80–89.

Shaw, R (2013) *The activist's handbook: winning social change in the 21st century*. 2nd ed. London: University of California.

Sheperd, J (2019) Timeline: the road to nurse registration in the UK. [Online] Available: www.nursingtimes.net/news/centenary-of-the-register/timeline-the-road-to-nurse-registration-in-the-uk-07-10-2019/ [Accessed: 12 May 2022]

Smith, D, Thomson, K, Bambra, C and Todd, A (2019) The breast cancer paradox: a systematic review of the association between area-level deprivation and breast cancer screening uptake in Europe. *Cancer Epidemiology*, 60: 77–85.

Snee, H and Goswami, H (2021) Who cares? Social mobility and the 'class ceiling' in nursing. *Sociological Research Online*, 26(3): 562–580. https://doi.org/10.1177/1360780420971657

Snee, H, White, P and Cox, N (2020). 'Creating a modern nursing workforce': nursing education reform in the neoliberal social imaginary. *British Journal of Sociology of Education*, 42(2): 229–244. https://doi.org/10.1080/01425692.2020.1865131

St. Christopher's (2023) Dame Cicely Saunders. [Online] Available: www.stchristophers.org.uk/about/damecicelysaunders [Accessed: 3 March 2023]

Stavropoulou, A, Rovithis, M, Sigala, E, Pantou, S and Koukouli, S (2020) Greek nurses' perceptions on empathy and empathic care in the intensive care unit. *Intensive and Critical Care Nursing*, 58: 102814. https://doi.org/10.1016/j.iccn.2020.102814

Stewart, A (2016) *Basic statistics and epidemiology: a practical guide.* 4th ed. CRC Press.

Subu, MA, Wati, DF, Netrida, N, Priscilla, V, Dias, JM, Abraham, MS, Slewa-Younan, S and Al-Yateem, N (2021) Types of stigma experienced by patients with mental illness and mental health nurses in Indonesia: a qualitative content analysis. *International Journal of Mental Health Systems*, 15(77). https://doi.org/10.1186/s13033-021-00502-x.

Sweeney, A (2022) Advocacy and activism: inspiring undergraduate nursing students. *Journal of Nursing Education*, 61(11): 660.

Tarrow, S (2022) *Power in movement: social movements and contentious politics.* Cambridge: Cambridge University Press

Taylor, J, Marland, G, Whitford, H, Carson, M and Leece, R (2022) Isolation and marginalization: exploring attrition of men in preregistration nursing programs. *The Journal of Nursing Education*, 61(4): 179–186. https://doi.org/10.3928/01484834-20220209-02

Taylor, Y, Lawrence, M and Andreasen, MB (2021) CILIA-LGBTQI+ comparing intersectional lifecourse inequalities among LGBTQI+ citizens in four European countries CILIA-LGBTQI + Comparing Intersectional Lifecourse Inequalities among LGBTQI + Citizens in Four European Countries Scotland Policy Brief. [Online] https://strathprints.strath.ac.uk/75572/1/Taylor_etal_CILIA_2021_Compaing_intersectional_lifecourse_inequalities_among_LGBTQI_plus_citizens.pdf [Accessed 3 August 2023]

Terry, L and Bowman, K (2020) Outrage and the emotional labour associated with environmental activism among nurses. *Journal of Advanced Nursing*, 76: 867–877. https://doi.org/10.1111/jan.14282

Tilburgs, B, Vernooij-Dassen, M, Koopmans, R, Weidema, M, Perry, M and Engels, Y (2018) The importance of trust-based relations and a holistic approach in advance care planning with people with dementia in primary care: a qualitative study. *BMC Geriatrics*, 18(1): 1–11. https://doi.org/10.1186/s12877-018-0872-6

UK Government (2013) Report of the Mid Staffordshire NHS foundation trust public inquiry. [Online] Available: https://www.gov.uk/government/publications/report-of-the-mid-staffordshire-nhs-foundation-trust-public-inquiry [Accessed: 16 June 2023]

UK Government (2018a) Chapter 5: inequalities in health. [Online] Available: www.gov.uk/government/publications/health-profile-for-england/chapter-5-inequality-in-health [Accessed: 3 March 2023]

UK Government (2018b) Chapter 6: wider determinants of health [Online] www.gov.uk/government/publications/health-profile-for-england/chapter-6-social-determinants-of-health [Accessed: 18 February 2023]

UK Government (2019) Mental health: environmental factors. [Online] Available: www.gov.uk/government/publications/better-mental-health-jsna-toolkit/2-understanding-place [Accessed: 12 November 2022]

UNISON (2019) UNISON the union for registered nursing. [Online] Available: www.unison.org.uk/at-work/health-care/representing-you/nursing/ [Accessed: 19 June 2023]

United Nations Development Programme (2022) Human development report 2021/2022. United Nations Development Programme. https://hdr.undp.org/system/files/documents/%0Aglobal-report-document/hdr2021-22pdf_1.pdf [last accessed 31 October 2022]

Universities UK (2020) Tackling racial harassment in higher education. [Online] Available: https://www.universitiesuk.ac.uk/sites/default/files/field/downloads/2021-08/tackling-racial-%0Aharassment-in-higher-education.pdf [Accessed: 1 May 2022]

Valdez, A (2021) Words matter: labelling, bias and stigma in nursing. *Journal of Advanced Nursing*, 77(11): e33–e35.

Van Bortel, T, Wickramasinghe, ND, Morgan, A and Martin, S (2019) Health assets in a global context: a systematic review of the literature. *BMJ Open*, 9(2): e023810. https://doi.org/10.1136/bmjopen-2018-023810.

Van Rickstal, R, Vleminck, A De, Engelborghs, S, Versijpt, J and Van den Block, L (2022) A qualitative study with people with young-onset dementia and their family caregivers on advance care planning: a holistic, flexible, and relational approach is recommended. *Palliative Medicine.* https://doi.org/10.1177/02692163221090385

Vancea, M and Utzet, M (2017) How unemployment and precarious employment affect the health of young people: a scoping study on social determinants. *Scandinavian Journal of Public Health*, 45(1): 73–84.

Vinje, HF, Langeland, E and Bull, T (2017) Aaron Antonovsky's development of salutogenesis, 1979 to 1994. In: Mittelmark MB, Sagy S, Eriksson M, et al. (eds) *The handbook of salutogenesis.* Cham: Springer. Chapter 4. [Online] Available: www.ncbi.nlm.nih.gov/books/NBK435860/. doi: 10.1007/978-3-319-04600-6_4

Wade, DT and Halligan, PW (2017) The biopsychosocial model of illness: a model whose time has come. *Clinical Rehabilitation*, 31(8): 995–1004. https://doi.org/10.1177/0269215517709890

Wall, S (2010) Critical perspectives in the study of nursing work. Journal of Health Organisation and Management, 24(2): 145–166.

Watson, J (2020) Nursing's global covenant with humanity: unitary caring science as sacred activism. *Journal of Advanced Nursing*, 76: 699–704. https://doi.org/10.1111/jan.13934

Wenger, E (1998) *Communities of practice: learning, meaning, and identity.* Cambridge: Cambridge University Press.

Whitley-Hunter BL (2014) Validity of transactional analysis and emotional intelligence in training nursing students. *Journal of Advances in Medical Education and Professionalism*, 2(4): 138–145.

Wittenauer, J, Ludwick, R, Baughman, K and Fishbein, R (2015) Surveying the hidden attitudes of hospital nurses' towards poverty. *Journal of Clinical Nursing*, 24(15–16): 2184–2191. https://doi.org/10.1111/jocn.12794

Woolnough, H, Fielden, S, Crozier, S and Hunt, C (2019) A longitudinal investigation of the glass-ceiling in nursing. *Journal of Managerial Psychology*, 34(2): 96–109. https://doi.org/10.1108/JMP-02-2018-0093

World Health Organisation (2018) Health inequities and their causes (who.int)

World Health Organisation (2019) Nursing. [Online] Available: www.who.int/topics/nursing/en/ [Accessed: 8 April 2022]

World Health Organisation (2021) COVID-19 and the social determinants of health and health equity. [Online] Available: www.who.int/publications/i/item/9789240038387 [Accessed: 22 June 2023]

Wright Mills, C (1959) *The sociological imagination.* Oxford: Oxford University Press.

Zappas, M, Walton-Moss, B, Sanchez, C, Hildebrand, JA and Kirkland, T (2021) The decolonisation of nursing education. *Journal for Nurse Practitioners*, 17(2): 225–229. https://doi.org/10.1016/j.nurpra.2020.11.006

ZareKhafri, F, Torabizadeh, C and Jaberi, A (2022) Nurses' perception of workplace discrimination. *Nursing Ethics: An International Journal for Health Care Professionals*, 29(3): 675–684.

Zauderer, CR, Ballestas, HC, Cardoza, MP, Hood, P and Neville, SM (2008) United we stand: preparing nursing students for political activism. *The Journal of the New York State Nurses Association*, 39(2): 4–7.

Index